"I love the new book *The New You: A Guide to Better Physical, Mental, Emotional, and Spiritual* . . . small steps that every person can . . . tual or physical breakthrough i . . . are looking for the big miracle . . . one answer to solve all their problems. This exciting book focuses on small steps . . . many small steps . . . to transform your life."

Elmer L. Towns, cofounder and vice president,
Liberty University

"Are you tired, worn down, discouraged, and longing for a vibrant life—a new you? Then this book is the prescription you need. Nelson Searcy and Jennifer Dykes Henson have compiled a simple, yet comprehensive, list of biblical principles anchored in scientific fact that when applied energizes the tired, rejuvenates the worn down, and invigorates the discouraged. Because of God's design for life, if you do what this book teaches, you cannot avoid a healthier and happier life."

Timothy R. Jennings, MD, DFAPA, psychiatrist and author
of *The Aging Brain: Proven Steps to Prevent Dementia
and Sharpen Your Mind* and *The God-Shaped Brain: How
Changing Your View of God Transforms Your Life*

"*The New You* is like a handbook for life. The content is clear, concise, and compelling. And Nelson and Jennifer write in a style that is straightforward, biblical, and highly practical. Your life will be better if you read and do what this book says."

Lance Witt, founder, Replenish Ministries

"Having no vision for your life should be alarming. However, having a big vision with no plan is senseless. This book will help you cultivate both! I love what Nelson and Jennifer have done because they've made complicated concepts incredibly approachable. You're going to want to keep this book near you for the rest of your life."

Clay Scroggins, lead pastor, North Point Community Church

"Searcy has taught us how to launch, grow, and sustain healthy churches, and now he and Henson share practical tips for attaining and maintaining healthy lives. *The New You* proves a timely book, as Christians are recognizing in increasing number the call to offer our bodies as living sacrifices (Rom. 12:1)."

Matthew C. Easter, assistant professor of Bible,
Missouri Baptist University

"The best book in a long time about how to balance spiritual *and* physical health! Searcy and Henson give an easy-to-follow plan for improving health while growing your spiritual life. Keep this book on your nightstand, in your car, or in your bag to consult it often and learn how physical health and spiritual growth were intended to work together."

Bob Whitesel, DMin PhD, award-winning author of 13 books, coach, consultant, and speaker on church health and growth at ChurchHealth.net

"Progress, not perfection! This approach to life keeps me sane and moving in the right direction. It is also what makes *The New You* such a valuable tool for making the most of your wellness. This book combines helpful biblical insights with practical small steps for moving forward in your wellness. My favorite thing about these small steps is they are realistic and doable. Read and apply this book and your total person will be transformed!"

Steve Reynolds, pastor of Capital Baptist Church in Annandale, Virginia, and author of *Bod4God: Twelve Weeks to Lasting Weight Loss*

"Personal health has the potential to be a troublesome and turbulent issue for many persons. In this book Nelson Searcy and Jennifer Dykes Henson truly offer 'a new perspective on God's purpose for our health and wellness' hardwired in an understanding of who we are in relationship to God. That makes it a refreshing and eye-opening read. Their practical and frank confrontation of the questions and unhealthy habits we often have encourages truthful reflection on how we serve as ministers and Christians. This is balanced brilliantly with the small steps to change, which provide motivation and are nonthreatening for persons who can become overwhelmed by just thinking about getting healthy."

Dwight Fletcher, founder and senior pastor, Transformed Life Church, Kingston, Jamaica

"I am forever grateful for my relationship with Nelson Searcy. I first came into contact with Nelson about nine years ago through his books and resources for churches and pastors. I decided to join his coaching network. Best decision I ever made! At that time I had been the pastor of the church I planted for nineteen years. We were a small church of about one hundred people. Since that time, through the coaching I received from Nelson, our church has grown to a church of over five hundred people, hired multiple staff, and built a building that enabled us to reach over 1,200 people this past Easter. We became a healthy, growing church. But the hard truth is—I was not a healthy pastor. I was overweight, out of shape, stressed out, and headed for an early grave. Two years ago, I finally decided to put into practice the principles that Nelson shares in this new book, the same principles that he has been living and sharing with me through coaching. Nelson is right, it really is the small things, done consistently over time, that make a huge impact in every area of life. In the past two years I've lost over eighty-five pounds and kept it off. I have more energy than I've ever had and I'm healthier than I've ever been. I cannot wait to share this book with you! You really are one small step away from a brand new you! Thank you, Nelson! My wife and family thank you! My church thanks you! I thank you!"

Pastor Chris Rollins, Coastal Community Church,
Charleston, South Carolina

"Nelson has been my friend and role model for ministry for nearly thirty years. I have witnessed him excel in every area of life from school to family life to church leadership. The principles that have helped him to be a good friend, husband, father, and pastor are shared in *The New You* in order to take you from an average life to an abundant life!"

Michael A. Jordan, pastor, Mount Vernon
Baptist Church, Axton, Virginia

"It's been said, if you want to know the health of a family, a church, or an organization, put a thermometer in the leader's mouth. In *The New You*, Nelson and Jennifer not only give the reader a checkup but they also give strategies for improving the most important areas of life. If you desire greater energy, clearer thinking, and spiritual vitality, this is the book for you."

Brian Moore, lead pastor, Crosspointe Church Anaheim

"This book will strengthen your life, regardless of your faith. Nelson applies his systematic, biblical, and practical approach to all areas of health. You will walk away stronger mentally, spiritually, physically, and emotionally. From the first chapter to the last, you will find big and small ideas you can use now. Don't wait, buy this book now."

Jimmy Britt, lead pastor, Rocky River Church,
Charlotte, North Carolina

"Nelson and Jennifer have done it again! Having known Nelson for over a decade, I have personally benefited from the teachings in this book. I recommend this book to everyone! And I think it would be a great book for small group study too."

"*The New You* is actually about *reclaiming* YOU! The YOU God envisioned . . . the YOU God created . . . the YOU God loves. In addition to physical health, Nelson and Jennifer delve into the spiritual, emotional, and mental dimensions of what makes for a healthy YOU. And that's where *The New You* really shines. Their holistic approach to your health provides insights galore and, at the end of each chapter, simple and specific strategies to help YOU reclaim more of what God intended for YOU all along!"

"Wholeness and healing are at the top of God's priority list. By clearly explaining the biblical principles that point to full health, the authors make human wholeness not only understandable but, through a series of small steps, doable."

the
new
you

A GUIDE TO BETTER PHYSICAL, MENTAL, EMOTIONAL, AND SPIRITUAL WELLNESS

NELSON SEARCY
JENNIFER DYKES HENSON

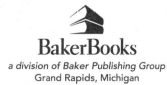

BakerBooks
a division of Baker Publishing Group
Grand Rapids, Michigan

To you, reader:

For having the courage
to seek God's best
in every area of your life.

Published by Baker Books
a division of Baker Publishing Group
PO Box 6287, Grand Rapids, MI 49516-6287
www.bakerbooks.com

Printed in the United States of America

Library of Congress Cataloging-in-Publication Data
Names: Searcy, Nelson, author.
Title: The new you : a guide to better physical, mental, emotional, and spiritual
    wellness / Nelson Searcy and Jennifer Dykes Henson.
Description: Grand Rapids : Baker Publishing Group, [2019]
Identifiers: LCCN 2018030086 | ISBN 9780801093302 (pbk. : alk. paper)
Subjects: LCSH: Peace of mind. | Self-help techniques.
Classification: LCC BF637.P3 S43 2019 | DDC 158.1—dc23
LC record available at https://lccn.loc.gov/2018030086

In keeping with biblical principles of creation stewardship, Baker Publishing Group advocates the responsible use of our natural resources. As a member of the Green Press Initiative, our company uses recycled paper when possible. The text paper of this book is composed in part of post-consumer waste.

g green press INITIATIVE

19 20 21 22 23 24 25   7 6 5 4 3 2 1

contents

acknowledgments

Nelson Searcy: My ongoing journey toward the new you, toward a comprehensive healthy lifestyle has been a rocky one. It all started in 1989, as a freshman in college, when I become a follower of Jesus. That decision kicked off an ongoing journey toward spiritual health. As life unfolded, the continual challenges of marriage, parenting, leading growing organizations and my own personal struggles pushed me to seek solutions for my mental and emotional health. I was a little late to the game—I finally started to get serious about my physical health in my mid-thirties, but better late than never. So I have been on the new you journey for quite a while and am healthier for it. My hope is that the thoughts and principles contained in this book will help you as much as they have helped me along the way.

It is not an overstatement to say that this book would not have happened without the obsessive commitment of Jennifer Dykes Henson. Jennifer and I have worked together on over a dozen books, but this one has been exceptionally dependent on her passion and dedication. It's an honor for me to be her coauthor on this book. Jennifer, her husband Brian, and their family all model the new you lifestyle. Jennifer, thank you!

I would also like to thank Steve Reynolds, who is referenced several times in these pages, for his impact on my thinking about health, especially mental and physical health. Steve is the pastor of Capital Baptist Church in Annandale, Virginia (Metro DC), and the author of several books. Search him online and pick up everything he has written. You won't be sorry.

There are so many others who provide support to my writing. The list of shout-outs includes, but is not limited to, Kerrick Thomas and Jason Hatley from The Journey Church; Sandra Oliveri, Seth Stone, and Raelyn Garriga from Church Leader Insights; and my most trusted advisors and friends, Jimmy Britt and Michael Jordan. There are so many others I could name, so please forgive me for providing only the short list.

Of course, it is my family that stands above all. During the year this book will be released, my wife and I will celebrate our twenty-fifth wedding anniversary. This milestone is known as the silver anniversary—though my wife deserves more than a silver medal for her commitment to me. Pray I find just the right gift! Likewise, my son, Alexander, will become a teenager this year. That may be the bigger prayer request! Kidding aside, I offer my deepest and ever-growing love to Kelley, and my ongoing love and appreciation to Alexander and the Christian young man he is becoming.

It has been a pleasure to work with the fine folks at Baker Books once again. This project was birthed in the vibrant mind of Chad Allen and then carried forward by Brian Vos, Colette Kischner, Robin Turici, Abby Van Wormer, and Brianne Dekker. I know there are many others at Baker Books whose names I don't know, who work hard behind the scenes as well—so thanks to everyone in acquisitions, editorial, publishing, and especially the frontline sales team. You all have my deepest appreciation!

Jennifer Dykes Henson: When I was just out of college, newly married, and working for Dr. Charles Stanley, I had the opportunity to sit in on some training sessions with Jordan Rubin, author of *The Maker's Diet* and founder of Garden of Life. The biblical truths I learned about health and wellness in those sessions set me on a path that changed the course of my own overall health, and ignited a passion that is culminating in the pages of this book. So first and foremost, I have to thank Jordan Rubin for his work, and for his willingness to pour the lessons of his own journey into others. I should also thank Dr. Stanley and the team at In Touch Ministries for opening the door to that connection.

My partnership with Nelson Searcy over the last thirteen years has been nothing short of incredible. I am continually humbled and excited to be involved in the magnificent work God is doing through him. *The New You* has been a true labor of love—one we are both passionate about and excited to bring to the world. I am honored to coauthor this book with someone so keyed into helping people everywhere achieve their full potential for God's glory. Nelson, thank you for inviting me into The Journey–Manhattan offices for that first meeting so many years ago and for all the ways you've encouraged our partnership to grow and evolve since. Each year—and each book—is more fun than the last!

Thanks to my husband, Brian, for being a constant well of love and encouragement and for continually challenging me to live a life worthy of the work I've been called to. And to my two young daughters, Isabelle and Ivey-Grace, my life's goal is to engage in the world in a way that will make you proud and that will model for you the fullness of life that Jesus offers us all. You are my inspiration for every word, for every breath.

Finally, thanks to God for once again giving me the opportunity to engage in meaningful work that will, hopefully and prayerfully, influence the lives of those who find it in their hands for the better.

introduction

Though no one can go back and make a brand new start, anyone can start from now and make a brand new ending.

Carl Bard

Therefore, since we are surrounded by such a huge crowd of witnesses to the life of faith, let us strip off every weight that slows us down, especially the sin that so easily trips us up. And let us run with endurance the race God has set before us. We do this by keeping our eyes on Jesus, the champion who initiates and perfects our faith.

Hebrews 12:1–2

Growing up, I (Jennifer) spent time at the beach every summer. Riding ocean waves with my dad was one of my favorite ways to pass the hot, salty days. We would wade out into the water, wait for the perfect little swell, and bodysurf it in to the shore. Over and over again, for hours at a time, we'd let one wave after another carry us to the sand.

One thing about playing in the ocean always caught me off guard. After we had been out in the water for a while, I would look back at the beach and not be able to find our big blue beach umbrella with my mom sitting beneath. Without realizing it, we had drifted so far from our starting point that we couldn't even see it anymore. The undertow had pulled us a long way in a direction we didn't even realize we were going. So we had to hit pause, walk up the beach until we found where we had started, and dive in again.

It wasn't until I was an adult with a family of my own that I realized undertows aren't just for the ocean. They exist in everyday life as well. Extra weight, low energy, a constant sense of anxiety . . . these things converged to teach me that drift is a real and active force. If we aren't intentional, our health and wellness slowly start to slip away as our days get busy with the demands of family life, work concerns, and messy relationships. The pull is so subtle that sometimes we don't even recognize it until months or years have passed. One day we wake up, look around, and think, *How did I get here?*

Nelson's Story

A few years ago, I wasn't living my best life. As a pastor, I had spent my entire career building God's church, but in the meantime, I had let my own health fall by the wayside. Sometime in my thirties, I began putting on a few extra pounds every year. I began sleeping less in the name of productivity and wrestling with more stress. I was on a downhill slope toward obesity, burnout, and ineffectiveness.

But, honestly, I wasn't that concerned. I was too busy to be concerned. Sure, I wanted to look and feel a little better, but doesn't everyone? That wasn't enough incentive to change my behavior. Besides, really getting healthy seemed overwhelming. The scale had ticked into intimidating territory, and I could feel myself struggling physically, spiritually, emotionally, and mentally. But habits are strong, and my unhealthy ones continued to direct my path.

Then came the breaking point. I became a father. When my son was born, I couldn't ignore what I was doing to myself any longer. I remember thinking, *I'm not going to be able to chase him around and enjoy his childhood if I don't get myself together.* That realization opened a floodgate. It led me to begin considering everything else my unhealthy lifestyle choices would keep me from doing in the future if I didn't make a change—things like being an engaged husband, fulfilling my role as a pastor effectively, simply living with contentment and enthusiasm. So I made a decision to stop being carried by the current of bad habits, tastes, and temptations. I took a hard look at the truth about my health and wellness and put a plan in place to get back to the fullness of life God had in store for me.

What's God Got to Do with It?

As we each (Nelson and Jennifer) set out on our individual journeys toward health and wellness, we began to understand a transformational truth: God has a plan for our health. He has a plan for yours. Your body and ours are the living, breathing, and walking around temple of God's Spirit. That reality has implications for how we care for ourselves physically, spiritually, emotionally, and mentally. Our skin, bones, and fleshy guts are home to the Most High. That is a humbling thought, isn't it?

As they say, the truth will set you free. A new, correct perspective on God's purposes for our health and wellness is a game changer. (We will explore that perspective in detail in the pages ahead.) After all, if God has entrusted us with these earthly vessels—not to mention all the work and plans he has for us while living in them—then where do we get off trashing them by eating what we want and sitting around letting them atrophy? Where do we get off neglecting sleep, harboring bitterness, and putting off the healing practice of prayer? (Maybe you don't do these things—we are speaking from personal experience here.) How can we rationalize treating ourselves so poorly that we can't fully engage in our Creator's purposes for us each and every day?

> "This means that anyone who belongs to Christ has become a new person. The old life is gone; a new life has begun!" (2 Cor. 5:17).

This goes a step further for those of us who are followers of Jesus. If you are a Christian, God has declared that you are a new creation in Christ. Scripture teaches that when you committed yourself to Jesus, you became a new person, fully and completely: "This means that anyone who belongs to Christ has become a new person. The old life is gone; a new life has begun!" (2 Cor. 5:17).

But even though we have been deemed new creations in Christ, many of us aren't living that way. Instead, we are frustrated, overweight, short on time, low on energy, dealing with chronic lifestyle-related health issues, stressed about work and family, unable to say yes to God's plans, and not experiencing fulfillment. For too many Christians, health issues—whether physical, spiritual, emotional, or mental—have become a stumbling block to living the abundant life God intends. Too many of the people filling American churches each weekend aren't able to experience life to the fullest because they are struggling with their physical bodies, their minds and emotions, and their daily relationships with God. Can you relate?

Here is some great news: walking in the reality of your new life in Christ doesn't hinge on trying harder or doing better. First and foremost, it is about surrendering to the fullness of your transformed identity in him (more on this in chapter 9)—and then doing your part to live out that fullness in every aspect of your daily life, which is what we will concentrate on in the pages ahead.

God wants us all to live full, active lives, accomplishing the things he put us here to do. He wants us to be free to live and love well. We have a responsibility to cooperate with him to make that happen.

Life is too short and too precious, and God has invested way too much in us, for us to squander our potential and let poor lifestyle choices hold us back from all he has in store.

Maybe the story your life is telling today isn't the story you want it to tell. Maybe you aren't where you expected to end up when you waded into the ocean of adulthood, and you realize it is time to look around, trudge up the beach, and dive in again. If that is you, you are not alone. It is never too late for change. By picking up this book, you have

> *God wants us all to live full, active lives, accomplishing the things he put us here to do.*

taken a small step toward a brand-new life. As you will see in the pages ahead, small steps are powerful—more than powerful actually. They are life changing. They have changed our lives, and we are certain they can change yours too.

Finding Your Starting Point

How do you feel today? Do you feel healthy? Do you feel strong and energetic? How are you doing spiritually? Are you walking in deep relationship with God? How about emotionally and mentally? What is going on in your heart and soul? Are you living out the life God has in store for you, or is that life being sidetracked by poor health in a specific area?

The first small step in the journey toward the new you—toward complete health in every area—is recognizing where you are. Before we get started, take a minute to think about your overall health and wellness. Rate yourself from 1 (lowest) to 10 (highest) in each of the following areas:

_____I am a healthy weight.
_____I eat and drink in a way that nourishes my body.
_____I walk at least ten thousand steps every day.

17

_____I have good, authentic friendships in my life.

_____I volunteer regularly.

_____I spend time seeking God daily.

_____I have forgiven the people in my life who have hurt me.

_____I get seven to nine hours of sleep every night.

_____I manage stress effectively.

_____I am intentional about choosing thoughts that benefit me.

These numbers represent your starting point. If they are low, don't be discouraged. Be excited by the opportunity for growth. If your numbers are strong, that is great. As you work through these pages, focus on how you can make them even stronger. Whatever your starting point may be, God will find you there as you commit to getting healthier and displaying his excellence to an onlooking world.

Small Steps to the New You

Small, incremental steps are the key to transitioning from an unhealthy lifestyle to a healthy one, the key to stepping into the fullness of the new you. Don't think you have to undergo an instant extreme makeover to get where you need to be. Just focus on minor improvements every day, every week, and every month. Over time, you will be amazed at the cumulative effect of your small efforts.

> *Small, incremental steps are the key to transitioning from an unhealthy lifestyle to a healthy one, the key to stepping into the fullness of the new you.*

What if you could improve your health by just 10 percent over the next six months? What if you could improve it by 10 percent more the following six? That would make you 20 percent healthier this time next year than you are right now. If you could do that again the following year, you'd be 40 percent healthier two years from now. Small changes to your lifestyle can get you there. You don't have to be intimidated by anything discussed in the pages ahead. Just take in what works for you and make the changes that will help you get to where you know you need to be.

Beginning in chapter 3, we will be suggesting "Small Steps to the New You" at the end of each chapter. These small steps will help you start making simple changes to your lifestyle. You can work through them at your own pace as you read, or you can take "The Small Steps Challenge," a four-month challenge found at the back of the book that will lead you to incorporate specific small steps into your life each month. This approach may work well if you are reading *The New You* with others as part of a group study. Either way, the small steps we suggest will work together over time to revolutionize your health, taking you from feeling overweight, sick, stressed, tired, and average to being excited about life, eager to face every day, and ready to take on all that God has for you in the time you have left before he calls you home. How you approach these steps is up to you.

By being intentional about how you live today, you can do your part to ensure that you will be living your best life for all your tomorrows.

Our friend Dave Ramsey often talks about how being willing to live like no one else now will allow you to live like no one else later. Dave is a financial expert, so he is speaking in terms of how you view and handle money. But the same truth applies to health. If you are willing to make small changes now—changes that many others are not willing to make—you can live healthier for your entire life rather than suffer from the predictable results of unintentional living. You can avoid so many of the problems associated with excess weight, poor diet, lack of sleep, and high stress. You can sidestep much of the mental and emotional strain caused by poor thought patterns and poor relational practices. By being intentional about how you live today, you can do your part to ensure that you will be living your best life for all your tomorrows.

The Life You Have Imagined

Imagine what life would look like if you woke up in the morning rested and energized, if you ate in a way that fueled your body instead of making you feel overly full and sluggish, if you could slide on those jeans in your closet and feel good about the way you looked instead of feeling a quiet desperation about the passage of time and the unruliness of your body.

Imagine what life would look like if you didn't need medications and caffeine to keep you going, if problems with your family members didn't dominate your thoughts, if you were proud of how you shaped your days and of your contributions to your work and to the people around you.

Imagine what life would look like if you felt a sense of deep connection with God, if you were surrounded by others who knew you well and could help you through anything life threw your way, if you felt as if you were right on course with the greatest plan for your life.

All this and more is possible. You can live the life that now you may only be able to imagine. We wrote *The New You* to help you get there.

> Now all glory to God, who is able, through his mighty power at work within us, to accomplish infinitely more than we might ask or think. (Eph. 3:20)

20

small steps
to the new you

1

whose you are

Opening Up with God about Your Health

The reason why many are still troubled, still seeking, still making little forward progress is because they haven't yet come to the end of themselves. We're still trying to give orders, and interfering with God's work within us.

A. W. Tozer

Don't you realize that your body is the temple of the Holy Spirit, who lives in you and was given to you by God? You do not belong to yourself, for God bought you with a high price. So you must honor God with your body.

1 Corinthians 6:19–20

As a teenager, I (Nelson) spent some time speaking at young entrepreneur conferences around the country. Thanks to that circuit, I had the privilege of working alongside the late Zig Ziglar. A great Christian businessman and leader, Zig spoke eloquently about matters of vision, change, work, and commitment. One thing Zig used to often say has stuck with me through the years. "Character gets you out of bed; commitment moves you to action . . . and discipline [enables] you to follow through."[1]

Character, commitment, and discipline—the ability to move from where you are in life to where you want to be will flow from these three things. All intentional change is born out of character, anchored in the commitments you make, and achieved through discipline.

Your character drove you to pick up this book. Something inside you is longing to live life at a higher level. Maybe you can feel stress, sickness, or anxiety tugging at your shirtsleeve, and you know it is leading you down a path that should be avoided at all costs.

> *All intentional change is born out of character, anchored in the commitments you make, and achieved through discipline.*

Discipline will determine how well you follow through with the small steps we suggest—the steps that will help you realign your overall health and wellness with God's best plan for you. You will learn a great deal in the pages ahead about living to your full health potential, but how well you apply what you learn is completely up to you. No one else can change your life for you.

That leaves commitment. The commitments you choose to make in your life shape your path through this world. If you look back over the years, you can probably recognize a handful of commitments that have determined where you are today. Maybe you made a commitment to go to one school over another, and that decision led you to your current life situation. Perhaps you made a commitment to marriage, or you may still be hoping to make that commitment one day. If you have children, you made a commitment to love and raise them well. Each one of these is a life-changing commitment. Stepping out of the status quo and deciding to reclaim your health and vitality is also a life-changing commitment, one we hope you will make.

Three Key Commitments

When you have all areas of your health under control, you are free to live life to the fullest. To get started, choose to embrace the following key commitments that are foundational to becoming the new you:

- surrender your health to God
- stop making excuses
- start taking small steps toward change

These commitments form the basis of your ability to build a life marked by complete health and wholeness. We will look at the first commitment here and the other two in the chapters to follow.

Surrender Your Health to God

Here is a game-changing truth for you to consider: your body wasn't created for your own gratification; it was created for God's glory. But if you are like most people, you treat your body as if it is yours to do with as you please. You are quick to gratify your own tastes, preferences, and whims. But the reality is that your body was made both *by* God and *for* God.

> *Your body wasn't created for your own gratification; it was created for God's glory.*

First Corinthians 6:13 says, "[Our bodies] were made for the Lord, and the Lord cares about our bodies." You probably intuitively understand that God made your body, but maybe you have never thought of it as being made *for* him. If your body was made for the Lord, and he cares about your body, doesn't that mean you should care about your body too?

This is an area where most people—Christians in particular—need to flip the lens. Too often, we use God as the ultimate excuse for letting our health slide. We run our bodies down, fill them with disease-causing foods, let them atrophy from lack of movement, and then call it God's will when we get sick. We fill our minds with toxic thoughts, neglect healthy relationships with other people, fail to engage with God regularly, and then blame him when we wind up lonely and anxious.

The truth is that pursuing excellence in every area of our health is a way to honor God. His sovereignty is not an excuse to live any old way we want to live because he is going to work it out in the end; instead, he is the beacon calling us to live in a way that shines his brilliance to others. Keeping ourselves in good health is really an act of stewardship.

Good Health = Good Stewardship

Again, your body is not your own. It has simply been entrusted to you for a period of time. You are called to steward your health in the same way you steward your money, your time, and your relationships. As Rick Warren wrote in *The Daniel Plan*:

> This life is preparation for our next life, which will last forever in eternity. God is testing you on earth to see what he can trust you with in eternity. He is watching how you use your time, your money, your talents, your opportunities, your mind, and yes, even your body. Are you making the most of what you've been given? God isn't going to evaluate you on the basis of the bodies he gave to other people, but he will judge what you did with what you have been given.[2]

Have you ever thought about having to stand before God and give an account for how you cared for yourself—for how well you ate, how active you were in an effort to stay healthy, how intentional you were about managing your stress and your emotions to avoid negative health consequences? That is a scary notion, isn't it?

Most of us have never thought that deeply about our physical stewardship responsibility. But it is not too late to start. No matter what kind of health you are in this very minute, it is not too late to surrender your body—to surrender every aspect of your physical health and well-being—to God.

> Don't you realize that your body is the temple of the Holy Spirit, who lives in you and was given to you by God? You do not belong to yourself, for God bought you with a high price. So you must honor God with your body. (1 Cor. 6:19–20)

Start by having a conversation with him. Talk to God about your current health. If you haven't been taking care of yourself, repent of that. Ask God to help you be a good steward of the body he has entrusted to you. Only then, working from the foundational understanding that your body is not your own but his, can you forge ahead into the complete health he wants you to have. (For more on talking with God through prayer, flip to chapter 19.)

We will take a look at the second commitment—stop making excuses—in the next chapter.

2

drop the excuses

Shifting Focus from Difficulties to Benefits

Ninety-nine percent of failures come from people who have the habit of making excuses.

George Washington

Don't copy the behavior and customs of this world, but let God transform you into a new person by changing the way you think. Then you will learn to know God's will for you, which is good and pleasing and perfect.

Romans 12:2

Most of us are all too willing to latch on to the first excuse we can find to explain why our health is out of our control. Here are a few excuses specifically related to physical health:

- I'm just big-boned.
- I don't have time to work out.

- Since God is in control, he will take care of my body.
- I have an issue that makes losing weight impossible.
- I don't like the taste of healthy foods.
- Obesity, diabetes, and heart disease run in my family. They are genetic.

That last one reminds me of a joke I heard recently. An overweight man goes to his family doctor for a checkup. When the doctor shows concern over his weight, the man says, "Doc, the problem is that obesity runs in my family." The doctor replies, "No, the problem is that no one in your family runs!"

The excuses that fill our minds make us believe that we are at the mercy of things beyond our control. So we throw up our hands, convince ourselves that we are doing okay compared to the next person, and forge ahead with life, excuses firmly in place. Even if we can recognize the pattern of blame shifting, it is hard to break because—let's face it—being a victim takes the responsibility off our shoulders. We feel better about ourselves and have an easier time justifying the poor health choices in our lives if we can blame our current health situation on something other than our own daily decisions.

But no matter how much we try to outrun it, we can't get away from the truth that the apostle Paul so clearly levied in a letter he wrote to some friends thousands of years ago: "Do not be deceived: God cannot be mocked. A man reaps what he sows" (Gal. 6:7 NIV).

If you sow seeds of poor health into your life, poor health is what you will end up with. But the good news is that the truth works both ways. If you are intentional about sowing seeds that lead to good health, you will reap good health. If you sow seeds necessary for good relationships, you will reap good relationships. If you sow seeds of rest and restoration, you will experience less stress and less fatigue. If you sow seeds of connection with God, you will experience more of his presence. You get the idea.

Sowing good seeds looks a lot like taking responsibility for your life. It looks a lot like taking a hard look at where you are and where you want to be and deciding to do what needs to be done to bridge the gap. It is refusing to make excuses and choosing instead to make better choices—choices that lead to health and wholeness and to the life you want to be living. And, again, it is never too late to get started.

Debunking the Two Most Common Excuses

When you cut through all the excuses we are all guilty of using to justify our poor choices and bad behavior, most of them can be filed under two main categories: "I don't have time" and "I'm too tired." Let's look at what is really behind each one.

"I Don't Have Time"

A lack of time is the number one excuse people offer up for neglecting their health. Unfortunately for the excuse makers, it is never a legitimate claim. We are all busy. There is always something else on the to-do list that has to be taken care of right away. But we would suggest that no matter how busy your life is, you will always find time for what you consider to be most important.

Do you have time to get quiet before God each day? Do you have time to spend with your kids? Do you have time to put in an extra hour at work on that big project? Do you have time for that show on Netflix? Of course you do, because you understand the importance of those things (well, maybe not the last one). Likewise, when you understand the importance of being proactive about your health—and hopefully that won't be at the point of a life-or-death crisis for you—you will find the time to do it. Staying healthy is not a question of time; it is a question of priorities.

Still, most of us love this excuse because it makes us sound self-sacrificial. When we don't have time to eat well or work out because we are busy taking care of our kids, working long work-weeks, or investing in the relationships in our lives, well, that is just the price we pay for being responsible to our obligations, right? Wrong. This is nothing more than a righteous-sounding excuse for not taking care of ourselves.

In reality, eschewing your responsibility to practice healthy habits today means that more of your time will be occupied by health problems tomorrow. Going to doctors' appointments, waiting for prescriptions to be filled, and continuously checking your sugar level and blood pressure take a great deal of time out of your schedule. Those are precious hours spent away from your family and your work. Better to make time for healthy living now than to be forced to spend time (and money) dealing with health problems down the road.

Staying healthy is not a question of time; it is a question of priorities.

Once I (Nelson) committed to making exercise and healthy eating part of my routine, I became addicted to the results. What they do for me physically, mentally, emotionally, and spiritually is hard to overstate. Thanks to prioritizing my health, I am now more efficient with my time and better able to be there for the people I had been using as an excuse. I have a clearer mind and more energy to tackle every day's work. Healthy living is an investment of time, not an expenditure, and one that seems to multiply the hours exponentially.

"I'm Too Tired"

Unhealthy foods combined with a lack of exercise is a recipe for constant tiredness, which makes this excuse a self-perpetuating one. If you play the tired card, remember this: the biggest reason you are so tired is because of your unhealthy lifestyle. The longer you justify this kind of lifestyle, the more tired you are going to be—which will make the excuse even harder to break free from.

31

The only answer is to be intentional about taking a first step toward health. Make a healthy meal even though you are tired. Go for a walk even if you don't feel like it. Turn off your phone and get to bed a little earlier. Over time, with consistent effort, you will have more and more energy, and this excuse will begin to evaporate.

Shifting Focus

Excuses are nothing but a by-product of wrong focus. They come from concentrating on the obstacles to a healthy lifestyle rather than on the benefits of good health. Instead of dwelling on how hard changing your bad habits will be, shift your attention to all the ways being healthy will transform your life for the better. When you have a big enough why, the how won't seem so intimidating. Here are just three of the best benefits of a healthy lifestyle:

Don't let excuses rob you of your opportunity to live the life you were created for.

- *Good health will help you make the most of your life.* Since God went to such lengths to design the details of your body (Ps. 139), you should want to take full advantage of what he can do through it while you are alive. When you run it down with unhealthy foods, a lack of exercise, and massive doses of stress, you block that opportunity. Rather than making the most of your one, precious life, you trade it in for a counterfeit version of God's best. Poor health choices will limit your potential and likely shorten your time on this earth, but taking care of yourself will allow you to fully engage in the life God has in store for you.

- *Good health will help you feel better and be more productive each day.* If you get your health on track, you will have

32

more energy every day. You will have fewer aches and pains. Your mind will be clearer. You will look better and be happier. You will be able to work harder and connect with the people in your life with more enthusiasm. Doesn't that sound like a great way to live? Don't let excuses rob you of your opportunity to live the life you were created for.

- *Good health will give you a new opportunity to worship God.* Since your body is the temple of God (1 Cor. 6:19–20), taking care of yourself well is a form of worship. Intentional good health brings God glory. Don't miss the opportunity you have to worship your heavenly Father and show his goodness to a watching world by being an example of excellent, vibrant health every day.

Now let's take a look at the third key commitment to getting your health on track: start taking small steps toward change.

3

small steps

A Simple Process for Becoming the New You

If you do what you've always done, you'll get what you've always gotten.

Henry Ford

Since, then, we do not have the excuse of ignorance, everything— and I do mean everything—connected with that old way of life has to go. It's rotten through and through. Get rid of it! And then take on an entirely new way of life—a God-fashioned life, a life renewed from the inside and working itself into your conduct as God accurately reproduces his character in you.

Ephesians 4:21–24 Message

One of our favorite sayings is "There is no elevator to success. You have to take the stairs." When it comes to health, physical health in particular, plenty of people buy into elevator philosophies: pills, powders, fad diets, extreme exercise plans . . .

you name it. Why? Because making an ongoing lifestyle change sounds a little too much like taking the stairs—and it will probably require walking some literal ones.

We want the quick fix. But quick fixes always lead to short-term results, followed by a face plant right back into the condition we were in before we started. We may find success for a few weeks, or a couple of months, but it won't be sustainable. Then the yo-yoing begins.

Quick fixes always lead to short-term results.

Think, for example, about that popular diet that comes around under a new name every few years—you know, the one that advocates losing weight by cutting out carbohydrates. Sure, that elevator will take you to a skinnier floor, but only as long as you stay on it. The problem is that kicking carbohydrates for life is not only unrealistic but also nutritionally unsound. Your body needs healthy carbohydrates to function effectively. As soon as you start eating them again, the weight returns with a vengeance and you are back on the ground floor, if not in the basement. Not to mention, the amount of meat consumed on these plans is directly and inarguably linked to many health issues (more in chapter 5). And this is just one of the popular, quick-fix weight-loss plans out there.

The point is that health-related shortcuts will only put you farther behind in the long run. The only way to get and stay physically well is to commit to an ongoing healthy, balanced lifestyle and then get started.

An Ancient Search for Excellence

As I (Nelson) began my own journey toward health, I found myself particularly interested in the life of Moses. Moses was the leader of over a million people. He lived a life of vision and momentum, leaving a legacy that still lives on thousands of years after his death. He was a guy intent on walking in the fullness of life God wanted to give him. And choosing to take responsibility for his health enabled him to do just that. Look how he is described at the end of his life: "Moses was 120 years old when he died, yet his eyesight was clear, and he was as strong as ever" (Deut. 34:7).

Moses was as strong as ever at 120 years old, while most of us feel the wear and tear of age by our early forties, if not before. Sure, we live in a different time than Moses did, but we can draw some pretty accurate conclusions about how he took care of himself from what Scripture tells us about his lifestyle. We know he stayed active by walking a lot (as documented throughout Exodus), he ate only the portion of food provided for him each day (Exod. 16:4), and he communed intimately with God (Exod. 33:11).

I want to live a long life. I want to live to be at least one hundred years old, just like Moses. But I don't want to live my later years being sick, lost in dementia, and dependent on someone else to take care of me. I want to be healthy, strong, and productive until my last day. I want to be in good physical health, of sound mind, and able to make a positive difference with my life for as long as possible. Just like Moses, I want to honor God with the health choices I make so I can experience all God has for me. How about you?

Living a long, happy life won't happen by accident. It won't happen if you just put your health on autopilot and hope for the best. Finishing well will require intentionality. Moses engaged in a way of life that, along with God's help and grace, allowed him to live to a vibrant old age. You can too. Engaging in this way of life means adopting a lifestyle of complete health—one that honors God and God can honor in return. It means sowing good seeds so you can reap good results. To get there, you have to focus on making ongoing adjustments in four specific areas:

- physical health
- spiritual health

- emotional health
- mental health

Just imagine what life would look like if you were living up to your full potential in each of these areas. How would you feel? What would you do? Whom could you influence?

Embracing the New You

You don't have to look far for advice on how to live a healthier life. There is an excess of information about how to get healthy, how to drop weight, how to have more energy, how to sleep better, how to reduce stress, how to, how to, how to . . . There is so much information—and misinformation—out there that it is hard to figure out what is even true.

Maybe you have read all the health books. Maybe you feel you know everything you need to know to get healthy, but you just can't make anything stick. Or maybe this is the first book about health and wholeness you have ever picked up. Maybe you have come to the end of your rope. You want to change, but you don't know how. You try to make tweaks here and there—you cut carbs for a while, you decide to work out and do so a few days in a row, you start a new morning devotional and do well with it for the first week, you commit to going to bed early until that football game or awards show on television keeps you up—but then all of a sudden you are back at square one, back to your old ways, still desperate for something new, promising yourself you will start again on Monday. Enter the apostle Paul once again: "I want to do what is right, but I can't. I want to do what is good, but I don't. I don't want to do what is wrong, but I do it anyway" (Rom. 7:18–19).

You and Paul have something in common. We all do, because this is the human condition.

Why Is Staying Healthy So Difficult?

Why is it so difficult to make the changes we want to make? The desire is truly there. Our intentions are good, and yet we fail time and again. That is because three major things work against us.

We Are Wrestling with the Flesh

As long as we live in these human bodies, we will be engaged in a struggle with our flesh. We may know what we should do, but there is always going to be resistance to overcome.

> *As long as we live in these human bodies, we will be engaged in a struggle with our flesh.*

Our bodies will want to sleep later, even though we know we need to get up and exercise. Our bodies will want our favorite comfort foods, even though we know smarter choices will lead to better health. Our hearts will want to hold on to unforgiveness, even though we know letting go will heal us. The struggle is real. Here is a little more of what Paul had to say about it:

> So the trouble is not with the law, for it is spiritual and good. The trouble is with me, for I am all too human, a slave to sin. I don't really understand myself, for I want to do what is right, but I don't do it. Instead, I do what I hate. But if I know that what I am doing is wrong, this shows that I agree that the law is good. So I am not the one doing wrong; it is sin living in me that does it. (Rom. 7:14–17)

The tug-of-war inside us won't go away as long as we are living, so we have to learn to overcome it.

An Enemy Wants to Rob Us of God's Best

Whether we acknowledge it or not, an enemy is continually working against us. We are engaged in never-ending spiritual warfare. When we don't understand that reality, we are much more susceptible to it. We are prone to think that our own weakness is the only thing keeping us bound. But this is not the case. Our struggle is bigger than ourselves. As Jesus said, "The thief's purpose is to steal and kill and destroy. My purpose is to give them a rich and satisfying life" (John 10:10). In Scripture, this thief, the devil himself, is also known as the tempter (Gen. 3). His goal is to keep God's people from living the lives God has in store for them—and he can do this in very subtle ways.

One of the enemy's greatest tools for keeping us bound to average, mediocre living is an attack on our health and wellness. If he can keep us sick, tired, stressed, and bitter, he is essentially thwarting our ability to fully live out God's purposes. Nothing would make him happier. As Peter wrote:

> Stay alert! Watch out for your great enemy, the devil. He prowls around like a roaring lion, looking for someone to devour. Stand firm against him, and be strong in your faith. Remember that your family of believers all over the world is going through the same kind of suffering you are. (1 Pet. 5:8–9)

If you are stuck in the rut of poor health in any area, not living an abundant life and not working to your full potential, the enemy is thrilled. He is getting his exercise doing a happy dance because you are compromised; you are not being as effective and influential as you could be.

Even though the enemy is constantly scheming, we are capable of standing firm against him. We can win the battle and walk into all God has for us.

Even though the enemy is constantly scheming, we are capable of standing firm against him. We can win the battle and walk into all God has for us. We just have to recognize and resist the devil's ploys. As James 4:7 says, "So humble yourselves before God. Resist the devil, and he will flee from you."

Spiritual warfare is nothing to be taken lightly. Whether you are familiar with the concept or not, it has implications for your life day in and day out. If you are skeptical, don't take our word for it. We invite you to dig in and do your own research. (For a list of resources, go to NewYouBook.com.)

We Have Been Taught to Compartmentalize Our Health and Wellness

We address our health in an ad hoc sort of way. We don't really consider how this workout plan or that stress-relief tactic will work for our overall well-being, or if it will be beneficial for us long term. We are usually more concerned about how we can drop fifteen pounds before our friend's birthday bash or how we can squeeze a few more hours out of the day without waking up tired.

The truth is that health and wholeness cannot be compart-mentalized. You are not just your physical body. You are not just your heart, your mind, or your emotions. Every part of your being either supports or puts drag on every other part. That is why it is impossible to be truly healthy in any one area if you are unhealthy in others. Paul acknowledged this truth in another letter to early believers: "Now may the God of peace make you holy in every way, and may your whole spirit and soul and body be kept blameless until our Lord Jesus Christ comes again" (1 Thess. 5:23).

Paul's words allude to the four areas of health we will be discussing in the pages ahead: physical health, spiritual health, emotional health, and mental health. You will never be able to achieve full health unless you address all four of these areas. Your overall health is the sum of the health of your parts.

The key to improving your health in each area is simply to get started. Draw your line in the sand and step over it into a new life. Change is possible. We know you are ready for it because this book is in your hands. You sense a better way of living is waiting for you, and it is. There is an abundant life, a life of wholeness.

And it can be yours. All you have to do is start taking small, daily steps that will produce big rewards in the long run. In other words, start taking small steps to the new you.

Small Steps to the New You

1. Surrender your health to God. With what you have read in mind, pray something like this:

   Dear God, I know that you made me. You created my body, my soul, and my spirit. You created me for your glory. I am sorry for the ways I have mistreated myself in the past. I am sorry for the excuses I have made for poor health choices and poor habits. I give this path to health and wholeness over to you. Please walk it with me. Please keep me focused on your truth, and help me to choose excellence every day. Thank you for creating me to live an abundant life, to do good work, and to love others well all my days. I surrender every aspect of my health to you now. Thank you for all you are going to do in and through me. Amen.

2. Stop making excuses. What is the biggest excuse you make for why you are not where you want to be? Be honest with yourself. Don't be afraid to look that excuse in the face. When you know what it is, refuse to make that excuse anymore. If you find it creeping into your mind, stop the thought and replace it with the following: God is able to do a great work in me.

3. Start taking small steps toward change. Just picking up this book is a great step in the right direction. Tell someone you trust that you are reading it. Ask that person to hold you accountable to making healthy changes in your life.

4. Be intentional about the small steps in the chapters ahead. Turn to the back of the book and start "The Small Steps Challenge" on your own or with others.

small steps
to better
physical health

4

your secret sin

The Spiritual Impact of What You Put in Your Mouth

The religious lifestyle has long been considered a healthy one, with its constraints on sexual promiscuity, alcohol and tobacco use. . . . However, overeating may be one sin that [people] regularly overlook.

Kenneth Ferraro

Sodom's sins were pride, gluttony, and laziness, while the poor and needy suffered outside her door. She was proud and committed detestable sins, so I wiped her out, as you have seen.

Ezekiel 16:49–50

An unaddressed sin is undermining American Christians today—one we have come to accept as normal, even though it has the potential to derail us completely. It is not what you might expect—not an addiction to drugs, alcohol, or pornography, even though these struggles are very real for some. No, this issue is sneakier. It cloaks itself in a shroud of normalcy and engages us in a daily battle so subtle that many of us don't even realize we are at war.

This sin tiptoes into our days in the form of cakes and cookies brought to the office by well-meaning coworkers, large cups of sweet tea sweating in our car consoles on hot summer days, the weekend potluck table filled with creamy casseroles and fried fixings. It thrives thanks to our almost universal addiction to sugar, fat, and refined carbohydrates—to all those things that excite our taste buds, course into our bodies, make us feel good for a moment, and then leave us a little thicker around the middle, a little unhealthier than before, and a little less vibrant.

Have you guessed it yet? Yep, the sin that is tearing us down is gluttony. A glutton is commonly defined as "one given habitually to greedy and voracious eating," or as "one who eats to excess or who takes pleasure in immoderate eating."[1] Gluttony is so prevalent that it is almost invisible. Its signs and symptoms are accepted as a normal part of life. You may not think you have a sin relationship with food, and, sure, yours may not be as severe as the next person's, but if you have been raised in this country and consistently carry more weight than you'd like to, the odds are not in your favor.

Picking and Choosing

We in the American church are notorious for picking the sins we want to make a big deal out of and overlooking the ones that don't bother us so much. Gluttony is a classic case of that type of thinking. While it is just as much a sin as theft or pride or drunkenness, we have chosen to give it a wink and a smile as we drive through the fast-food lane and upsize our meals.

Can you imagine if a huge percentage of America's professing Christians were bound by drug addiction or involved in illicit affairs? The church would collapse. We would be called hypocrites and run out of every town. Biblically and culturally, we all understand just how unacceptable those sins are.

But while gluttony is also unacceptable biblically, it has become an accepted vice culturally. We embrace this sin. And not only do we embrace it but we also like to get together to commit it. While we hold ourselves and others accountable for more obvious, less accepted sins, we don't have any problem stuffing ourselves to excess and then parading our bulging bodies—the public evidence of our private downfall—around for all to see. Some would say that we are testing God. Actually, Scripture says, "They stubbornly tested God in their hearts, demanding the foods they craved" (Ps. 78:18).

Sure, we have a hundred excuses for why our weight and health problems aren't our fault. We look to the ways and wisdom of the masses to justify our eating habits. Every weekend many of us promise ourselves we will start eating better on Monday. But when Monday rolls around, nothing has changed, so nothing changes. We fall into the pattern we are used to. We eat what we want, when we want, to the point of excess . . . and our enemy smiles.

Defending Our Indulgence

Some skilled biblical debaters use Scripture to try to argue their way around taking care of their bodies. They claim that, based on Scripture, we can eat whatever we'd like. They point to one passage in particular:

> "It's not what goes into your body that defiles you; you are defiled by what comes from your heart." Then Jesus went into a house to get away from the crowd, and his disciples asked him what he meant by the parable he had just used. "Don't you understand either?" he asked. "Can't you see that the food you put into your body cannot defile you? Food doesn't go into your heart, but only

passes through the stomach and then goes into the sewer." (By saying this, he declared that every kind of food is acceptable in God's eyes.) (Mark 7:15–19)

A close examination of this passage proves that dietary leniency is not really its point. The Old Testament is filled with specific dietary laws addressing what is okay to eat and what isn't. Most of these laws focus on clean versus unclean meats. Later, the book of Acts records a vision God gave to Peter in which he told Peter that all meats had been declared clean (Acts 10:9–16). Mark's account above sets the stage for that vision. Jesus is underscoring the point that God made to Peter: a person can't be defiled by what goes into their stomach—spiritually speaking, that is.

Many Christians cling to this passage, and to Peter's vision, to prove that they have permission to eat whatever they want to eat. "Food can't hurt me," they say. "God said I can eat anything I want, so pass me a fork." Unfortunately, this argument is based on complete misinterpretation. The vision God gave to Peter and Jesus's discussion in Mark are both making the point that we are no longer spiritually bound by dietary laws. Jesus abolished those requirements.

> *Paying attention to what God says about food gives us the greatest chance for excellent health.*

The verses are referring specifically to holiness in the eyes of God. By declaring all things clean, God said there are no longer direct spiritual consequences for eating something that was once considered off-limits. Thanks to that mandate, sticking to certain dietary guidelines no longer makes or keeps us holy. But (and this is a big *but*) that doesn't mean the wisdom contained within them for our physical health is null and void.

What is interesting is that most of the Old Testament laws concerning food coincide with what modern science tells us about the healthiest ways to eat. And why wouldn't they? God designed our bodies, designed food for them, and then put dietary boundaries in place for our own good. Paying attention to what God says about food gives us the greatest chance for excellent health. For example:

- Eat lots of fruits and vegetables (Gen. 1:29).
- Fish with scales and fins are healthier than sea scavengers (Lev. 11:9–11).
- Pigs don't digest the toxins they eat, so their meat isn't healthy (Lev. 11:7–8).
- Eat wholesome, life-giving breads (Ezek. 4:9).

And the list goes on. Take a look at what Rex Russell wrote in *What the Bible Says about Healthy Living*:

> The primary message of both the Old and the New Testaments is salvation; and salvation comes through the blood sacrifice of the Messiah, not through eating habits. Nevertheless, a large portion of the Scripture focuses on commands, ordinances and statutes that show us how to live on this carefully designed earth. Many of these passages pertain to subjects such as economics, law, government, interpersonal relationships, nutrition and health. The sacrifice Jesus made for our sins does not cancel the wisdom in these other teachings. As Paul said, they are still profitable.[2]

The foods we choose to eat can't influence our spiritual standing in God's eyes, but that reality has absolutely nothing to do with how those same foods affect our physical health. As Paul wrote, "You say, 'I am allowed to do anything'—but not everything is good for you. And even though 'I am allowed to do anything,' I must not become a slave to anything" (1 Cor. 6:12).

Have you become a slave to what you put in your mouth? It is easy to do—and it is even easier to justify in today's food culture. Let us ask another way: Are the foods you put in your mouth doing more to serve your immediate desires or your future dreams and goals? God wants you to make choices that will set you up for success down the road rather than just satisfy your appetite in the short term. He wants to produce self-control—the direct antithesis to gluttony—in you, through his Spirit. Galatians 5:22–23 says, "But the Holy Spirit produces this kind of fruit in our lives: love, joy, peace, patience, kindness, goodness, faithfulness, gentleness, and self-control."

The everyday choices you make to keep yourself healthy are so important, both to the quality of your life and to your ability to do all God has planned for you.

Be careful of letting others convince you that God isn't concerned with what you eat. You are his careful creation. You are his hands and feet on this earth. He wants to put you to good use and shine through you mightily. The everyday choices you make to keep yourself healthy are so important, both to the quality of your life and to your ability to do all God has planned for you.

Making excuses and using Scripture to justify the sin we love leaves us playing right into our enemy's hands. There is nothing he would rather do than convince us that God is okay with us overloading our bodies with foods that will eventually kill us. After all, when our bodies fail, then we are out of service. Let's decide to stop ignoring our own gluttony and get on with living a better life for the glory of God.

Small Steps to the New You

1. Take a hard look at the gluttonous habits you may have in your life. Decide to stop justifying them.

2. Acknowledge that God's understanding of your physical health needs surpasses your own.

3. Go to NewYouBook.com and listen to a message about breaking free from gluttony.

5

eating for life

*Three Small Shifts in Your Diet
That Will Make a Big Difference*

You have a clear choice. You can live longer and healthier than ever before, or you can do what most modern populations do: eat to create disease and a premature death.

Dr. Joel Fuhrman

So whether you eat or drink, or whatever you do, do it all for the glory of God.

1 Corinthians 10:31

A new baby always brings new perspective. If you have children, think about the moments right after they came screaming into the world. While you probably believed in the miracle of God's creation before, something about seeing a new life appear in front of you woke you up to just how incredible God is—and how much effort he has put into making each one of us.

Psalm 139:13–14 says, "For You formed my inward parts; You covered me in my mother's womb. I will praise You, for I am fearfully and wonderfully made" (NKJV). Wow. You are *fearfully and wonderfully made*. Do you feel like it? Do you walk through each day embracing that truth? You are a product of a generous, intelligent Creator who crafted you in his image. He gave you a beating heart and lungs to breathe.

Not only did he create you and me but he also placed us in a world specifically designed to sustain us in health and wholeness. He gave us food to nourish us and water to quench our thirst. He told us to get busy working the land. He told us that if we follow his ways, we will be blessed with long life (1 Kings 3:14). And many of our earliest ancestors—those who ate a more primitive diet and lived a more active lifestyle than we do—often lived to a vibrant, healthy old age.

> Most of the ailments filling our prayer request lists are reversible—better yet, altogether preventable—with some simple dietary changes.

Things look a little different today. Our collective health choices have put us on a downward spiral toward chronic illness and early death. A hundred years ago, lifestyle-related diseases such as diabetes, heart disease, and even cancer were rare. In many cultures—those that have never stopped eating the way generations before us did—that is still the case. Yet for those of us living in modern, westernized countries, these types of diseases have become commonplace.

Like fish in water, most of us have a hard time recognizing our own environment. We need a wake-up call. We need a paradigm shift. We need to grasp the fact that we are bringing so much of the pain of poor health on ourselves. Most of the ailments filling our prayer request lists are reversible—better yet, altogether preventable—with some simple dietary changes. The cliché is scientific truth: we are what we eat. And what we eat is killing us. It is time to get back to the basics and begin nourishing our bodies the way God intended. It is time to start taking responsibility for what we put in our mouths.

Back to Basics

What if you woke up tomorrow morning and found the car of your dreams sitting in your driveway? Imagine that an anonymous do-gooder heard that you had always wanted a Range Rover (or a Lamborghini, or a new, top-of-the-line Cadillac . . . whatever it may be) and decided to leave one parked where your old car sat the night before. How would you react? How excited would you be?

More to the point, how would you treat that car? I bet I can guess. You would keep it clean, you wouldn't let the kids eat in it, you would make sure it was serviced on time, and you would give it the premium fuel that the manufacturer meant for it to have, wouldn't you? There is no way you would risk hurting it by filling it with a lower grade of gas than it needed to function as it was supposed to. After all, not only would that be a slap in the face to the person who gave you the gift, but it would also keep you from being able to enjoy this dream come true at peak performance for as long as possible.

Amazingly, we all understand this concept when it comes to taking care of a car, but when it comes to our own bodies, we don't make the connection. Here is the reality: God gave you a fantastic gift. He gave you an intricately designed body, specially formed for the purpose of being his representative on this earth. He gave you breath to fill your lungs and a pumping heart to circulate your blood. He gave you a mind capable of more than you can fathom. He placed your soul inside this meticulously crafted vessel and handed it over to you as a gift. How are you treating it? Are you treating it as well as you would treat that car? What are you pouring into it on a daily basis to make sure it operates well for the long haul?

When you eat the foods that keep your body healthy, you are cooperating with God's best plan for your health. By taking responsibility for your food choices, you are being a good steward of the one and only body he has entrusted to you. Unfortunately, cultural norms and free will have thwarted God's best intentions for the majority of us—but it is not too late. You can get back to the health God wants you to have. You can work with him rather than against him by making better choices, starting today. God won't do this for you. To do so, he would have to go against the natural laws of cause and effect that he put in place. But if you do your part to be healthy, you can trust God to bless your efforts.

Part of the problem is that we overcomplicate things. God's prescription for health is pretty simple: eat the foods he created in the closest possible form to their original creation. In other words, eat an apple, not an apple fritter. Eat a piece of wild salmon, not a microwavable fish stick. As Jordan Rubin wrote in *The Maker's Diet*:

> Most Americans eat great quantities of food frequently, based on convenience. In fact, the entire fast food [industry has] flourished due to our fast-paced lifestyles. . . . Unfortunately, the Creator didn't design our bodies to operate at optimum levels on junk food, fast food, or prepackaged foods. His laws that govern our entire human nature, including our health, bring consequences when violated, whether or not we accept the fact that they are still in place.[1]

To reclaim your health and begin functioning the way God intended, you have to get back to his original plan for your eating habits. You have to get back to basics.

Here are three overarching guidelines that have the power to revolutionize your health and put you back on the path to wellness.

Eat Living Foods

Then God said, "Look! I have given you every seed-bearing plant throughout the earth and all the fruit trees for your food." (Gen. 1:29)

Living foods are the fruits, vegetables, beans, and grains God created specifically to fuel our bodies. They are made up of nutrients and enzymes specifically designed to work in connection with our bodies' systems to sustain health and energy. In their natural state, fruits, vegetables, beans, and grains are so nutritionally complex that many of the healthful compounds within them haven't even been identified. For example, a tomato contains more than ten thousand different phytochemicals, all of which work together to benefit the body.[2] The range and composition of these phytochemicals is so involved that scientists are still trying to identify the details of God's craftsmanship.

Then there is the other end of the spectrum. Processed, packaged foods can be considered dead foods. While living foods are foods that God made, dead foods are foods created or drastically altered (think potato chips rather than fresh potatoes) by humans. The name "dead foods" is appropriate because not only do they contain no living energy but they will also lead you down the fast track toward sickness and death if you eat enough of them. Just think about it: if something can sit on a supermarket shelf for months (even years) and still be considered safe to eat, there is obviously no life in it. Living things die. That food is nothing but a combination of chemicals and preservatives wrapped up in an appealing package and laced with sugar and salt to keep you going back for more.

The first key to taking responsibility for your health is to decide to start filling your plate with living foods. Eat fruits and vegetables. Eat beans and whole grains. Make sure your food choices include a lot of color—or, as it is sometimes said, eat a rainbow every day. Green, red, orange, and yellow fruits and vegetables will fill you with living energy and flood your system with the building blocks of superior health. When your diet includes large quantities of the living foods God made, you are not only staving off obesity and all its negative consequences but also proactively fortifying your cells against disease—particularly cancer.

In nutritional science circles, cancer has come to be known as a fruit and vegetable deficiency disease. "The *Journal of the National Cancer Institute* reported that men who ate three or more servings of cruciferous vegetables a week [such as broccoli and cabbage] had a 41 percent reduced risk of prostate cancer compared with men who ate less than one serving."[3] That is a huge percentage. When the same men added a variety of other vegetables to their diets, the risk went down even more.

If someone created a pill that slashed cancer risk by close to 50 percent, everyone in America would want to take it. The good news is that we can accomplish the same thing by being wise about what we put in our mouths. The bad news is we just don't do it. Why? Taste? Culture? Habits? These are all weak excuses for failing to cooperate with God to maintain our health.

Speaking of pills, many people think that if they take a multivitamin, they don't need to eat fruits and vegetables. While vitamins are an important part of a healthy lifestyle, no vitamin can duplicate the unique nutrient composition found in whole fruits and vegetables—a combination of synergistic elements (antioxidants, flavonoids, phytonutrients, etc.) that work in the body to minimize inflammation, destroy harmful cells, and boost health. Focus your energy on nutrient-rich foods, not isolated, scientifically extracted "nutrients." Good health doesn't come in a bottle or happen by chance; it is earned one bite at a time.

Good health doesn't ... happen by chance; it is earned one bite at a time.

Trade White for Whole Grain

Now go and get some wheat, barley, beans, lentils, millet, and emmer wheat, and mix them together in a storage jar. Use them to make bread for yourself. (Ezek. 4:9)

Perhaps you have heard the expression "If it's white, don't bite." This quirky phrase is grounded in truth. Refined carbohydrates, such as white bread, white rice, white pastas, and most baked goods, are one of the major culprits behind America's weight and sickness epidemic.

Not all carbohydrates are created equal. The carbohydrates found in fruits, vegetables, beans, and whole grains are known as complex carbohydrates and are essential building blocks of health. But the refined (read: processed) carbohydrates so prevalent today are dangerous beyond measure. They have had all the nutritional value stripped out of them. What remains is nothing but sugar—literally. When refined carbohydrates enter your body, they are converted directly into sugar, which is why they are responsible for so many obesity-related diseases.

Consider this study. Over a period of six years, scientists tracked forty-three thousand men whose diets were high in white rice, white bread, and white pasta. The participants had two and a half times the incidence of type 2 diabetes as those who ate high-fiber alternatives such as whole-grain bread and brown rice.[4] Type 2 diabetes is nothing to be taken lightly. It is the seventh leading cause of death in America[5]—and completely preventable. In addition to causing obesity and diabetes, these nutritionally defunct foods also lead to higher incidences of heart disease and many types of cancer.[6]

As you begin to fill your diet with more living foods, also be intentional about cutting out refined carbohydrates. Opt instead for whole-grain products. Whole-grain varieties retain the fiber and nutrients not found in refined carbohydrates, so they interact with your body in an entirely different way. One note of caution: be wary of breads and other baked goods that are simply labeled "whole wheat." They are often just white bread products with a little coloring added. Make sure you read the nutrition label and buy only products in which whole-grain components are first on the list of ingredients.

Limit Animal Protein

Do not mix with winebibbers, Or with gluttonous eaters of meat; For the drunkard and the glutton will come to poverty. (Prov. 23:20–21 NKJV)

Don't worry. We are not going to tell you that you have to become a vegetarian. But we are going to recommend that you begin practicing some significant moderation when it comes to the amount of meat you eat. To say that the amount of animal protein we all consume is significantly higher than that of generations past is a huge understatement—and this extreme increase is directly responsible for many of the health problems we struggle with today.

A hundred years ago, meat was more of a treat than a staple. Sunday dinner was special because it was usually the only meal of the week in which meat was served. These days, however, we have come to believe that a meal isn't complete unless it includes meat. As a result, most Americans are eating meat at least twice, if not three times, every day—and in large quantities at that.

This is problematic on a couple of levels. First of all, most forms of animal protein are high in saturated fat, and saturated fat intake is directly linked to the skyrocketing rates of heart disease and cancers we are facing in this country. Second, the more meat we fill up on, the fewer fruits, vegetables, and whole grains we are going to eat. We are trading the nutritional benefits contained in those foods for something that is not nearly as beneficial to our health. Writing about the findings of the China Project, the most comprehensive study ever done on the relationship between diet and disease, Dr. Joel Fuhrman, a leading specialist on disease prevention and reversal, noted:

> The data showed huge differences in disease rates based on the amount of plant foods eaten and the availability of animal products. Researchers found that as animal foods increased in the diet . . . so did the emergence of the cancers that are common in the West. Most cancers occurred in direct proportion to the quantity of animal foods consumed. . . .
>
> All animal products are low (or completely lacking) in the nutrients that protect us against cancer and heart attacks—fiber, antioxidants, phytochemicals, folate, Vitamin E, and plant proteins. They are rich in substances that scientific investigations have shown to be associated with cancer and heart disease incidence: saturated fat, cholesterol, and arachidonic acid.[7]

The amount of cholesterol and saturated fat that most of us consume from animal sources significantly outweighs the amount of healthful nutrients we consume from plant sources. This reality is leading us down paths of sickness and premature death much more quickly than any meat-loving American wants to admit. Fuhrman added:

> Never forget that coronary artery disease and its end result— heart attacks, the number one killer of all American men and women—are almost 100 percent avoidable. . . . Most of the poorer countries, which invariably consume small amounts of animal products, have less than 5 percent of the adult population dying of heart attacks. . . . The major risk factors associated with heart disease—smoking, physical inactivity, eating processed food, and animal-product consumption—are avoidable. Every heart attack death is even more of a tragedy because it likely could have been prevented.[8]

One of the wisest steps you can take in your journey toward health and wellness is to cut back on meat. That means both red and white meat. No, you don't have to eliminate meat altogether, but keeping the amount to less than 10 percent of your intake each week and filling that new gap with fresh vegetables, fruits, beans, and grains (not pasta and onion rings) will put you squarely on the path to incredible health.

Breaking the Addiction

These three tweaks to your diet are simple, but that doesn't necessarily mean they are easy. The way you eat today is the result of years of conditioning. There will be a learning curve while you retrain your taste buds to enjoy flavors you may not have been exposed to very much. You will probably experience a few withdrawal symptoms as you cut out refined carbohydrates and their sugary counterparts. Right now your body is addicted to those things, and the addiction has to be broken.

You can do this. The other side of the mountain is worth the effort it takes to get there. Aren't you ready to take control of your eating habits rather than letting them control you?

Small Steps to the New You

1. Add more colorful fruits and vegetables into a few of your meals this week.

2. Start reading nutrition labels on breads, pastas, and baked goods. Buy only products that are 100 percent whole grain.

3. Trade white rice for brown rice.

4. Try limiting your intake of meat to one meal a day.

6

avoiding common obstacles

How to Get Ahead
of What Could Hold You Back

Failure is not a single, cataclysmic event. You don't fail overnight. Instead, failure is a few errors in judgment, repeated every day.

Jim Rohn

Forgetting the past and looking forward to what lies ahead, I press on to reach the end of the race and receive the heavenly prize for which God, through Christ Jesus, is calling us.

Philippians 3:13–14

As you start down this path toward taking responsibility for your health, you are creating a new lifestyle—stepping fully into the new you. This isn't a quick fix. As with every journey worth taking, there are going to be a few setbacks. Don't let those discourage you. Progress, not perfection, is the goal.

If you blow your commitment at one meal, don't think of the whole day as shot. Start again with your next meal. Discouragement will try to set in, but don't let it. You may be tempted to quit, but be quick to shoot that temptation down. When the enemy tries to whisper defeat in your ear, refocus your attention on Jesus, the one who promises you can do all things through him (Phil. 4:13)—all things, including losing extra weight, ridding yourself of lifestyle diseases, and reclaiming your health for his glory.

Progress, not perfection, is the goal.

Common Obstacles

That said, a few obstacles are common to almost everyone who commits to changing the way they eat for the better. Knowing what those obstacles are and preparing for them in advance can help you stand strong when they threaten to throw you off balance. These are the ones that top the list:

- resistance
- emotional eating
- a lack of family support
- eating out

Let's take a look at each one in more detail.

Resistance

The unrelenting pull of the average, culturally acceptable (unhealthy) lifestyle is real and powerful. The resistance you feel when you start taking action toward a healthy lifestyle is a live, active force. Stephen Pressfield, in *Do the Work!*, has written in detail about resistance.

Resistance cannot be seen, heard, touched, or smelled. But it can be felt. . . . The more important a call or action is to our soul's evolution, the more Resistance we will feel toward pursuing it. Resistance's goal is not to wound or disable. Resistance aims to kill. Its target is the epicenter of our being: our genius, our soul, the unique and priceless gift we were put on this earth to give.[1]

Pressfield's words sound a lot like Jesus's description of the devil himself. "The thief's purpose is to steal and kill and destroy" (John 10:10).

The enemy of your soul is also the enemy of the purposes God has for you on this earth. He wants to kill you. Period. And he is hoping he can do that by your own hand. He wants to make you think you can't change your life. He wants to deceive you into believing a couple of unhealthy meals won't matter. He is trying to keep you traveling the path toward your own destruction. He is applying consistent, subtle pressure to get you to settle for your current state of being, to be okay with health that looks like everyone else's, to live a life that is lacking the abundance Jesus came to give you. But as James wrote so plainly, "Resist the devil, and he will flee from you" (James 4:7).

When the enemy tries to tempt you to go back to your old way of life, resist. When you feel tempted to grab an unhealthy meal out of convenience rather than take the time to eat something that will nourish your body, resist. As you get in the habit of opposing the enemy's schemes, he will turn his attention toward someone else. Resist the resistance.

Emotional Eating

We are all guilty of using food to make ourselves feel better. The comfort foods we know and love do a great job of helping us calm down when we are anxious and picking us up when we have had a rough day—or do they?

When you look to food to give you an emotional boost, you may get a momentary surge of pleasure from what you eat, but ultimately, you end up feeling worse. Not only are your problems still there but you also feel guilty about gorging. This can lead to a downward spiral of resignation and even more emotional eating.

Emotional eating is a common problem. A large percentage of people who struggle with overeating and excess weight are emotional eaters. We all live busy, stressful lives. (If that statement is not true of you, you are in the minority these days. Let us know your secret.) If you are like most people, you just want to sit down and decompress at the end of the day—and a bag of chips, a pint of ice cream, or dinner's leftovers often seem like the perfect couch companion. But when you allow yourself to eat out of emotional hunger rather than physical hunger, not only are you adding to your health problems but you are also failing to deal with the stress in your life productively.

To begin getting emotional eating under control, figure out what your most common triggers are.

To begin getting emotional eating under control, figure out what your most common triggers are. What situations or feelings make you want to reach for comfort food? Maybe you are triggered when you are under a great deal of stress, or maybe your trigger is nothing more than boredom or even just force of habit. Whatever your trigger, start taking intentional note of when your eating is driven by something other than hunger.

Then when you catch yourself reaching for food for the wrong reasons, pause. Tell yourself you are going to wait ten minutes before having that snack. Use those ten minutes to do something that may help you deal with your emotions in a healthier way. Go for a quick walk. Pick up a book. Connect with your spouse. Talk with God in prayer. When those ten minutes have passed, your urge to eat will likely have passed too—and you will have taken a step toward managing your emotions in a much healthier way.

A Lack of Family Support

Healthy lifestyle habits are much easier to adopt when everyone in your household is on the same page, but that is not always the way it works. You may find yourself a lone ranger in a house full of people who have no interest in changing. If that is the case, keep focused on why you are making the shift toward complete health and continue pressing toward your goal.

Your success may eventually have a major impact on the people you love. They may want to sit back and watch for a while, but when they begin seeing the changes in your body, your increase in energy, and your overall improved quality of life, they may want those things for themselves. They may start asking questions. For Christians, this process is a little like being a witness to an unbelieving world. Make the people around you so curious about the positive changes in your life that they will want to know what you know.

Practically speaking, if your family isn't with you on this, you may need to take some inconvenient steps to stay on track. If your spouse does the grocery shopping, make sure healthy items get put on the list and in the cart. Designate a separate area of the refrigerator for your healthy foods so you can get right to them without having to rummage through old temptations.

While going it alone in your home won't be easy, commit to carrying the torch. When you stay strong on your own, not only will you be better for it but your entire family will benefit as well. They may begin their own healthy journeys in their own time, and you will have been part of their catalyst rather than an enabler of ingrained mind-sets and habits.

Eating Out

Restaurant meals can be one of the worst enemies of a health-conscious lifestyle. But with a little preplanning and a handful of strategies for success, eating out can become part of your healthy routine rather than an excuse for slipping back into your old ways.

First of all, if you know you are going to be eating out, be intentional about choosing a restaurant that will have some healthy options. As much as it is up to you, avoid places where you will have a hard time finding something you will feel good about on the menu. Also try to avoid your old haunts, where familiar smells and ingrained habits may push you over the edge of temptation. You may be able to go back to those places one day and order with more wisdom, but don't put yourself in that position too soon.

If you are eating out with family, friends, or coworkers who want to go somewhere that doesn't offer good choices for you, don't be shy about suggesting an alternative. If they know you are committed to getting healthy, they will likely be more than willing to go somewhere different.

Once you are in a restaurant, keep these tips for success in mind:

- *Pray*. Before you order, have a quiet talk with God. Thank him for the changes he is making in your body and for the newfound health in your life. Ask him to help you choose a meal that will nourish the body he has given you. (Remember, surrender.)

- *Focus*. Focus your attention on the healthiest options on the menu. Don't even read about the burger and fries. Look for vegetables, hearty salads, and grilled dishes. And don't hesitate to ask your server how something is prepared. If you want to make a special request, go for it. Most restaurants are more than happy to work around dietary concerns.

- *Order first*. I know, I know, we are supposed to put others first. But when you are on a mission to get healthy and you are sitting in a restaurant with other people, make an exception. When the server is ready, be quick to order before anyone else does. That way you won't be tempted to change your order when you hear what those around you are having.

- *Eat less.* Portions in most restaurants arc out of control. Even if you order something healthy, there will probably be enough of it on your plate to feed you and the person next to you. Decide before the food hits the table that you are not going to eat it all. Get rid of the "clean plate club" mentality when it means eating two or three times more than your body needs. Consider asking for a take-out container as soon as your meal arrives, then set some of the food aside for later.

Progress, Not Perfection

Remember, setbacks are part of the process on this journey toward renewed health. Learning to navigate your world with an entirely new lifestyle will take some time and practice—that is okay. Take small steps every day. Be aware of the obstacles along your path. If you mess up, shake it off and start again. Get a little better week by week. And always keep reminding yourself "Progress, not perfection, is the goal."

Small Steps to the New You

1. Acknowledge the reality of resistance in your life—and resist it!

2. Take a ten-minute pause before snacking to make sure you are actually hungry.

3. Claim a corner of the refrigerator for your healthy groceries.

4. Choose restaurants that will have healthy options. You may even want to look at the menu online before you go so you know what your choices will be before you get there.

7

drink up

Water, Weight Loss, and How Much You Need

Pure water is the world's first and foremost medicine.

Slovakian proverb

The earth was formless and empty, and darkness covered the deep
waters. And the Spirit of God was hovering over the surface of
the waters.

Genesis 1:2

When you wake up in the morning and it is raining, do you
thank God for the downpour, or do you think, *Oh no.
I have to drive the kids to school in this!* Most of us lean toward
the latter, but really we should be praising God for the incredible
gift he is sending us—the gift of water.

Your brain and heart are 73 percent water. Your lungs are 83 percent water. Your skin is 64 percent water. Your muscles and kidneys

are 79 percent water. Even your bones are 31 percent water. Because you are composed largely of water, water is necessary for all your bodily functions. Without enough of it, your health will, well . . . dry up.

> *Because you are composed largely of water, water is necessary for all your bodily functions.*

Drinking like a Rock Star

Three-fourths of Americans walk around chronically dehydrated. Chances are, you are one of them. How often do you feel thirsty? When the feeling of thirst hits you, you are already dehydrated. Dehydration is a dangerous condition. Here are its most common symptoms:

- *Dry skin.* When your body is lacking water, it rations and prioritizes the little bit it does have. The brain and the heart are top priority, so the body makes sure to keep those two things hydrated. But other organs, including your skin (your body's biggest organ), suffer as a result. Despite all the lotions and creams you slather on to try to stay moisturized, dry skin is an internal problem.

- *High blood pressure.* While high blood pressure is mainly a result of poor food choices and other lifestyle issues, dehydration compounds the problem. Your blood is 83 percent water. When you aren't drinking enough water, your blood thickens and your heart has to work harder to circulate it. This complicates things for people with high blood pressure—and in some cases can even cause it.

- *Vocal cord damage.* A few months ago, I (Jennifer) went to a concert headlining one of today's most popular singers. I won't tell you his name, but if you keep your radio on all day, you will probably hear three or four of his songs. During the concert, every time he finished a song, he downed an entire bottle of water, practically in a single gulp. He is a smart guy. Water serves as a lubricant, like oil to a car. Especially if you sing or speak a lot, keeping your vocal cords hydrated is important. If you are having trouble sustaining your voice or have that dry-mouth feeling, start drinking (water) like a rock star.

The Well of Wellness

When there is enough of it, water accomplishes some amazing things in your body. Water

- gives you energy;
- regulates digestion by breaking down and flushing out waste;
- helps stabilize blood pressure;
- clears toxins from your body;
- reduces the chance of kidney stones;
- helps maintain your body's proper acid and alkaline balance;
- improves focus and mental acuity; and
- hydrates your skin and slows down the appearance of aging.

This is a pretty impressive list, isn't it? Sometimes we hear the objection, "I don't like water." Do you like being tired? Do you like having digestive problems? Do you like being constipated? Do you like high blood pressure? Do you like having an acid and alkaline imbalance? Do you like being overweight? Do you like having dried up, wrinkled skin? Do you like having problems with your kidneys and urinary tract? No? Time to drink some water!

70

Water and Weight Loss

If the above benefits aren't enough, consider this: drinking more water will help you lose weight. Any healthy lifestyle plan is going to focus on diet and exercise, but it must also include an emphasis on drinking large amounts of water. Consider these facts about water and weight loss:

- Initial weight loss is largely water loss. You need to drink plenty of water to avoid dehydration as those pounds drop away.

- Efficient calorie burning requires an adequate supply of water. Dehydration slows down the fat-burning process.

- Burning calories creates toxins that must be flushed out. Water is essential to ridding your body of the toxic buildup that must be eliminated.

- Dehydration causes a reduction in blood volume. A reduction in blood volume causes a reduction in the supply of oxygen to your muscles, which in turn makes you feel tired. You don't want to eat right and exercise when you are tired.

- Water helps maintain muscle tone and lubricates your joints. Proper hydration can help reduce muscle and joint soreness when you start becoming active.

- A healthy diet includes a great deal of fiber. Without adequate fluids, this necessary fiber can cause constipation.

- Drinking water with a meal helps you feel full and satisfied more quickly. If you are well hydrated, you will be more likely to eat only as much food as your body needs.[1]

71

Drinking more water will help you lose weight.

Since getting your weight under control is a major first step toward excellent health, you literally can't afford to push water aside. Once you get used to drinking it in large quantities, you will be glad you did. You will feel cleaner, clearer, and more alert. Your body will actually begin craving more and more water every day, and you will quickly realize that water is fine.

Small Steps to the New You

1. Start your day with water. Adopt the habit of drinking a full bottle of water first thing every morning. Doing so will rehydrate you after a night's sleep, wake up your system, and jump-start your metabolism for the day. Try putting a bottle of water in the bathroom where you shower and dress in the morning. Before you finish getting ready, finish that bottle of water.

2. Keep water close at all times. Carry a bottle with you in your car (if it is plastic, keep it in the shade) and have one handy in your bag. If you always have water within reach, you will be much more likely to stay hydrated—and to opt for it over sugary drinks.

3. Add lemon or some other fruit for flavor. Not only does this vary water's taste but most fruits also provide an alkalizing effect. Keeping your body properly alkalized is important to your overall health.

4. Drink only water when eating out.

5. Eat more fruits and vegetables. Most fruits and vegetables have significant water content. When you eat an apple, banana, squash, or carrot, not only are you getting essential nutrients and fiber but you are also getting water.

6. Replace sugary drinks with water. The sugar contained in sodas (diet sodas are no better), sports drinks, sweet tea, sweetened coffee drinks, and most store-bought juices is wreaking havoc on our bodies. Work toward replacing all the sugar-filled drinks in your diet with pure, clean water.

7. Drink half your body weight in water every day. Divide your weight by two. That is how many ounces of water you should aim for on a daily basis. As Don Colbert wrote in his book *The Seven Pillars of Health*:

> Picture a one-gallon container of milk and imagine it three-quarters full. If you are an average sized person, that's about how much water your body needs daily. If you weigh 120 pounds, you will need 60 ounces of water. If you weigh 220 pounds, you will need 110 ounces of water.[2]

8

made to move

The Easy Exercise
That Will Change Your Life

If we could give every individual the right amount of nourishment and exercise, not too little and not too much, we would have found the safest way to health.

Hippocrates

So I run with purpose in every step. I am not just shadowboxing. I discipline my body like an athlete, training it to do what it should. Otherwise, I fear that after preaching to others I myself might be disqualified.

1 Corinthians 9:26–27

Exercise. It is something we love to hate. Even if you are someone who enjoys exercise and understands the benefits for your body, maintaining the habit of exercise is not easy to do. Can I get a witness? Even so, it is a critical part of taking responsibility for your health.

Remember a few chapters ago when we mentioned that people often use Scripture to justify eating anything they want? Too many people try to do the same thing with exercise. You have no idea how many times I (Nelson) have heard people quote the following verse to me: "For bodily exercise profits a little, but godliness is profitable for all things, having promise of the life that now is and of that which is to come" (1 Tim. 4:8 NKJV).

"See?" they say. "The Bible says bodily exercise has little benefit. I need to spend my time focusing on more important things in my life." I can't blame them for clutching onto this excuse. I used to do the same thing. What I didn't consider, and what they don't either, is that the writer, Timothy, lived a drastically different lifestyle than we live today. In a normal day, just by walking everywhere he went and tending to his business, he was probably more physically active than many of us are in a typical two-week period. His life was full of built-in exercise; our lives are full of cars, elevators, desk chairs, and couches.

Once you hit your goal weight (and those new eating habits are fully integrated into your life), exercise becomes the key to helping you sustain your new healthy body for the long haul.

When you first begin your journey to take off extra weight, diet is the most critical factor. At first, exercise simply complements the changes you are making to what you put in your mouth. As you begin to drop pounds, exercise becomes more and more important. Once you hit your goal weight (and those new eating habits are fully integrated into your life), exercise becomes the key to helping you sustain your new healthy body for the long haul. This is good news for reluctant exercisers. It gives you a pass to get started slowly and ramp up—which is the wisest approach to a new exercise routine anyway.

Don't Just Sit There—Get Moving!

We were made to move. Our bodies were created for physical activity. God never intended for us to sit all day, overfilling our stomachs and letting our systems atrophy. But sedentary lifestyles have become the norm. The typical American is sedentary 60 percent of their waking hours.[1] This lack of physical activity is associated with a number of health problems, ranging from weight gain to osteoporosis to cardiovascular disease. Take a look at just some of the problems inactivity causes:

- People who are physically inactive have an increased risk of colon and breast cancer. One study showed a 40 percent decrease in cancer mortality in people who were physically active compared to those who were inactive.

- A recent study reported that for every two hours a person watched TV, the risk of type 2 diabetes increased by 14 percent. Physical activity helps prevent insulin resistance, the underlying cause of type 2 diabetes.

- Physical inactivity increases the risk of cognitive decline. One study reported a 50 percent reduction in the risk of dementia in older people who maintained regular physical activity.

- People who are sedentary have the highest rates of heart attacks. In the Nurses' Health Study, women who were physically active three hours or more per week (half an hour daily) cut their risk of heart attack in half.

- Strokes, which are often referred to as brain attacks, affect approximately 730,000 people annually and are linked to physical inactivity. Data from the Aerobics Research Center in Dallas, Texas, found that physically active men lowered their risk of stroke by two-thirds. And in the Nurses' Health Study, physically active women decreased their risk of stroke by 50 percent.

- Bones, like muscles, require regular exercise to maintain their mineral content and strength. Bone loss progresses much faster in people who are physically inactive.

- People who don't perform regular physical activity are more likely to become depressed. Physical activity is a good way to reduce mood swings and maintain a sense of emotional well-being.

- People who don't get regular physical activity are more likely to gain excess weight. One study showed that an hour of walking daily cut the risk of obesity by 24 percent.

- People who don't get regular physical activity have less efficient immune systems, which make warding off various diseases and illnesses such as colds and the flu more difficult.[2]

Are you convinced?

So the question becomes, How much exercise do we need to achieve the physical benefits we are looking for? Experts agree that the ideal amount of exercise we all need to maintain good health is seventy minutes, six days a week. If you aren't in the habit of exercising, that may sound like an impossible number to you. The best way to reach that amount is to start slowly with simple, consistent walking.

Walk for Wellness

Walking is the oldest physical activity known to humankind. Generations before us walked miles every day and didn't consider it exercise. Walking was just part of life; it was how they got from one place to another and went about their work. Our friend Steve Reynolds, author of *Bod4God*, has estimated that Jesus walked about fourteen miles a day.[3]

These days we have let a walking lifestyle slip by the wayside. Rather than walking a few extra steps, we drive around a parking lot for ten minutes, looking for a space closer to the door. If we would just park farther away, we could save time and get a little exercise to boot.

Most of us don't have to walk much on the job, so we have lost that opportunity too. Think about Adam in the Garden of Eden. The first task God gave him was to tend to the garden, which would have required a lot of walking. Now we may walk down the hall for a meeting or walk the aisles of the grocery store, but that is about the extent of it.

Not only is walking great exercise but it is also the perfect jumping-off point if you aren't used to getting much physical activity.

Not only is walking great exercise but it is also the perfect jumping-off point if you aren't used to getting much physical activity. Walking is cheap and convenient—and it will do wonders for your health. A brisk walk every day gets your blood pumping, raises your metabolism, and increases your body's ability to burn calories for up to twelve hours afterward.[4]

That said, you have to walk far enough to make it count. A healthy goal is ten thousand steps per day. In general, ten thousand steps equals just less than five miles. According to several recent studies, walking ten thousand steps every day leads to

- a 90 percent reduction in heart attacks;
- a 30 to 70 percent reduction in cancer rates;
- a 50 percent reduction in type 2 diabetes; and
- a 70 percent reduction in stroke rates.[5]

Walking ten thousand steps a day isn't nearly as difficult as you may think. When I (Nelson) first started trying to get more active, I was not in good physical shape. I was overweight and lethargic. As part of my plan to reclaim my health, I decided to take up running. The first time I put on a pair of sneakers and tried to run, I couldn't even make it sixty seconds. That first run turned into a walk around the block, and even that was hard! Nowadays, I try to run at least three miles most days of the week. On top of that, I have a goal to hit ten thousand steps throughout the rest of the day. I put a free pedometer app on my phone that tracks my steps (which I highly recommend; there are also many pedometer wristbands and watches on the market that can be helpful), and I am often amazed by how quickly those steps add up. You will be too.

Small, routine changes can help you work more walking into your life. What if you decided to take a ten-minute walk after lunch and dinner every day? Just schedule the time on your calendar. Walking for as little as ten minutes after a meal drastically changes your blood sugar level. What would you be doing instead? Sitting back down at your desk, with a food coma setting in? Sitting down on the couch to watch TV? Those are poor lifestyle choices that will keep you in the grip of poor health. Decide instead that you are going to walk around a parking lot or, if you are at home, around your neighborhood. Take the dog. It will be good for both of you.

As you begin to make walking a habit, you will naturally think of other ways to work in more steps on a daily basis. Here are a few ideas:

- Take the stairs instead of the elevator.
- If you live in an area where you can walk to have lunch or run some errands, do it. Limit your driving.
- Have something to discuss with a friend, family member, or coworker? Plan a "walk-and-talk" meeting. That is, take a

walk together to discuss whatever you need to discuss. Or walk while you talk to that person on the phone.

- Get up a few minutes early in the morning and take the dog for a walk.
- Ignore the most convenient parking space and choose to park farther away from your destination.

Set a goal to walk ten thousand steps every day. This small lifestyle change will pay huge dividends for your health and wellness.

When you feel ready, those ten thousand steps can become the foundation of an active lifestyle that includes other forms of exercise—maybe jogging, swimming, or biking. As you get stronger and healthier, experiment with different activities until you find a few you really enjoy. After a while, exercise won't be a chore; it will be something you look forward to, something that brings you energy and joy. Always remember that you were made to move. The more you move, the more you lose.

Small Steps to the New You

1. Download a pedometer app or buy a pedometer to track the number of steps you are walking in a day. Try to hit ten thousand.

2. Download a podcast or the audio version of a book you have been meaning to read and listen while you walk or work out.

3. Put your workout clothes and sneakers by the bed the night before and take a morning walk as soon as you wake up.

4. Need to call your mom? Plug some earbuds into your phone and take a walk around the neighborhood while you talk.

small steps
to better
spiritual health

9

living the fully engaged life

How to Assess Your Spiritual Health

Living a life fully engaged . . . is something most people plan to do, but along the way they just kind of forget.

Bob Goff

The eyes of the LORD search the whole earth in order to strengthen those whose hearts are fully committed to him.

2 Chronicles 16:9

Okay, so you know you need to eat healthier and get your body moving—and you have tried. You got psyched up to make healthy changes, you jumped in with both feet, and then bam. Before you knew it, you had ordered french fries and skipped two morning walks. You ended up frustrated, wallowed in the discouragement for a while, and then gritted your teeth and tried again. Wash, rinse, repeat. Just thinking about how many times you have started a new healthy eating or exercise plan only to crash and burn before noon of day three is probably pretty discouraging, right? We can relate.

Health cannot be compartmentalized. If you want to get healthy, you can't focus on just your physical body. You are so much more than that. You can't focus on just your mind or emotions either. Every part of your being is intertwined with every other part. Complete health will remain elusive until you take a holistic approach and address your entire self—body, mind, emotions, and spirit—as a whole.

If you aren't spiritually healthy, you will always struggle with your body, your mind, and your emotions.

That said, one aspect of the four towers above the others and ties them all together. Can you guess what it is? If you said spiritual health, go reward yourself with a green smoothie. Your spiritual health is the foundation on which a life of wholeness is built. If you aren't spiritually healthy, you will always struggle with your body, your mind, and your emotions. To get from where you are to where you want to be in any and every area of your well-being, you have to engage with God and take responsibility for your spiritual health. Doing so is the key to becoming the new you.

Engaging with God

Are you ready for some life-altering news? God is already fully engaged with you, and he is constantly inviting you to be fully engaged with him. When you take him up on the offer, he makes his strength available to you. Take a look at this Scripture passage: "The eyes of the LORD search the whole earth in order to strengthen those whose hearts are fully committed to him" (2 Chron. 16:9). God is looking for people who are ready to be fully committed to him. When he finds these people, he strengthens them.

What would your life look like if it were infused with God's strength? His strength would empower you to face the day with enthusiasm, to interact with other people joyfully, and to feel a sense of peace in the depths of your soul. His strength would energize you and give you the stamina you need to take care of your body well. His strength would help you face stressful situations with assurance. His strength would give you the courage to face emotional wounds that may be holding you back. God's strength is the linchpin to living a life that is full, happy, and healthy. Without it, you will always be searching, struggling, and faltering as you search for short-term fixes and temporary highs. Without him, you will never be fully healthy and whole.

God wants to give you his strength. In fact, he is eager to give it to you. He is already engaging with you, and he is inviting you to engage with him. God's level of engagement in your life is consistent. He doesn't waver. Take a look at these promises:

> You go before me and follow me.
>   You place your hand of blessing on my head.
> Such knowledge is too wonderful for me,
>   too great for me to understand!
> I can never escape from your Spirit!
>   I can never get away from your presence!
> If I go up to heaven, you are there;
>   if I go down to the grave, you are there.
> If I ride the wings of the morning,
>   if I dwell by the farthest oceans,
> even there your hand will guide me,
>   and your strength will support me. (Ps. 139:5–10)

Did you catch that? There is nowhere you can go where God is not engaged with you. He is both ahead of you and behind you. You can go to the highest mountaintop or the depths of the sea, and he will be there with you, with his hand of blessing on your head. Let that sink in. That is full engagement at its highest level.

The psalmist goes on to say that God knew you before you were born. As we have seen, you are intricately and wonderfully made. God knows your strengths and your weaknesses. He knows the good parts of your personality, and he knows your bad habits and quirks (see Ps. 139). He loves you anyway. He wants a relationship with you. He wants to be intimately involved in your life. He wants to do more in you, through you, and for you than you could ever ask or imagine.

> *At its core, the all-encompassing health we are striving for is nothing more and nothing less than complete health in Christ.*

This passage ends with, "Search me, O God, and know my heart; test me and know my anxious thoughts. Point out anything in me that offends you, and lead me along the path of everlasting life" (Ps. 139:23–24). In other words, "Okay, yes, God, I know you are engaged with me. Test me and show me where I am not engaged with you. Am I fully committed? Am I taking responsibility for my walk with you?"

Those are the questions we all have to answer as we set out on the path toward all-encompassing health. Why? Because at its core, the all-encompassing health we are striving for is nothing more and nothing less than complete health in Christ.

The Ultimate Demonstration of Engagement

Jesus is the ultimate demonstration of God's engagement in our lives. He is the visible representation of God's engagement. God sent Jesus to live a perfect life, to die on a cross for our offenses, and then to be raised from the dead—all so that we could be in relationship with him and have new life, both here and in eternity. John 3:16, the most popular verse in the Bible, illustrates this:

"For this is how God loved the world: He gave his one and only Son, so that everyone who believes in him will not perish but have eternal life."

If you want to know how far God is willing to go to demonstrate his love for you, look at Jesus. If you want to know how much God wants to be involved in your life, look at Jesus. If you don't believe the Bible can be trusted, I challenge you to consider all the other supporting evidence concerning Jesus and choose to look at him. He can stand up to all your doubts and questions.

God's engagement with us is clear. The question mark is our engagement with him. Scripture teaches that when you commit yourself to Jesus, you actually become a new creation. You become a new you, fully and completely. You are changed from the inside out—and not as a result of anything you have done or can do but because of what Jesus has done. Second Corinthians 5:17 says, "This means that anyone who belongs to Christ has become a new person. The old life is gone; a new life has begun!"

This is where wholeness begins. Walking in the reality of new life in Christ doesn't hinge on trying harder or doing better in any area. It is about surrendering to the fullness of your transformed identity in him and doing your part to live out that fullness in every aspect of your daily life.

With Jesus, you can go from struggling through your days to walking in step with the living God. This doesn't mean your circumstances will change immediately, but your daily decisions that influence them can. This doesn't mean there won't still be resistance, but you will have God's Spirit within you helping you push through. This doesn't mean the enemy won't still try to derail you, but you will be operating in the power of Jesus to overcome him.

How do you get there? How do you step into this new creation? How do you become the new you on a foundational level? First by saying yes to God's invitation to trust in his Son. If you haven't already done that, you can find out how and get many of your questions answered at NewYouBook.com. Then you make a decision every day to lean into the life God has for you. You can begin by doing the following:

- *Allow God to change the way you think.* "Let God transform you into a new person by changing the way you think. Then you will learn to know God's will for you, which is good and pleasing and perfect" (Rom. 12:2).

- *Choose to step away from old, unhealthy tendencies.* "Since, then, we do not have the excuse of ignorance, everything— and I do mean everything—connected with that old way of life has to go. It's rotten through and through. Get rid of it!" (Eph. 4:21–22 Message).

- *Develop new habits that will help you take hold of the life you want.* "Put on your new nature, created to be like God" (Eph. 4:24).

You enter into the life God has for you by first connecting with him through Jesus and then by taking responsibility for your spiritual health. As you do, you will begin to experience the fullness of life as the new you.

Taking Responsibility for Your Spiritual Health

How spiritually healthy are you? If we were able to sit down over a cup of coffee with you and we asked you to tell us about your walk with God, what would you say? Maybe you aren't sure about the whole God/Jesus/Christianity idea. You are skeptical, but curious, and just trying to figure things out. Or maybe you feel you are living in close connection with God. You are committed to his ways and trying to live a Christlike life every day. Wherever you are on the spectrum, take a step back and examine the areas where you are doing well and the areas where you need some improvement.

You have probably heard of the Gallup research organization. They have an arm that focuses on faith and Christianity. A few years ago, they studied tens of thousands of Jesus followers and determined that the people who are the most spiritually healthy, the most engaged with God, can answer true to the following statements. Think about each statement, and write a T (true) or F (false) next to each one:

_____My faith is involved in every aspect of my life.

_____Because of my faith, I have meaning and purpose in my life.

_____My faith gives me an inner peace.

_____I am a person who is spiritually committed.

_____I spend time in worship every day.

_____Because of my faith, I have forgiven people who have hurt me deeply.

_____My faith has called me to develop my given gifts and talents.

_____I will take unpopular stands to defend my faith.

_____I speak words of kindness to those in need of encouragement.[1]

_____I talk about my faith with those who are not yet Christians.

This list is a helpful gauge of your level of spiritual health. If you were able to answer with mostly Ts, that is great. Now rank each statement 1 to 10, with 1 being sometimes true and 10 being always true. Then you can work on bringing the numbers up on the ones that need the most work.

If you answered with mostly Fs, congratulations. We admire you for being willing to take the test and assess where you are in your spiritual health. Every F on the list is an opportunity to engage more with God. Ask him to go before you as you make a decision to begin taking on the attitudes and characteristics of Jesus and following his actions.

To move from where you are to where you want to be, you have to choose to engage with God and take responsibility for your spiritual health. This is the first step toward achieving overall health and wellness, which makes perfect sense if you think about it. As we have seen:

- God knit you together in your mother's womb (Ps. 139:13).
- Your body was made for God (1 Cor. 6:13).
- You were made to fulfill the work God has planned for you (Eph. 2:10).
- God wants to do more than you can imagine in you, for you, and through you (Eph. 3:20).

But the key to melding these truths together is to acknowledge who Jesus is and begin building your life on the foundation of his truth. Any time you sidestep your responsibility in this area, you will fall back into old habits and patterns in every area, and you will distance yourself from God. You can't live your life partially your way and partially God's way and hope to experience the benefits of full engagement. Only when you bring everything together under the umbrella of a single focus can you experience the power of a committed life. And that focus is becoming more and more like Jesus.

To move from where you are to where you want to be, you have to choose to engage with God and take responsibility for your spiritual health.

You can continue to go through life feeling as if you aren't quite where you want to be. You can continue to worry and to hold on to bitterness. You can continue to fall back when you have an opportunity to take a stand for your faith. You can continue to live tired, overweight, and sick. You can continue to wrestle with mediocrity. Or you can decide to step away from the frustration of a divided life and experience God's power at the highest level possible in every area, every single day. We say again, as we said in the beginning, the choice is yours. Jesus's brother James put it well in his letter to early believers: "Come close to God, and God will come close to you" (James 4:8).

Small Steps to the New You

1. Take the quiz in this chapter. Evaluate your answers. Jot down some ideas for how you could improve on each point.

2. Think about this question: Who is Jesus? If you don't know the answer, decide to find out. Don't rely on your past experiences or what people tell you. Do your own intellectually honest research about his life and ministry.

10

getting connected

Four Ways Church Can Help You
Become Your Healthiest Self

Wherever we see the Word of God purely preached and heard, there
a church of God exists, even if it swarms with many faults.

John Calvin

And let us not neglect our meeting together, as some people do,
but encourage one another.

Hebrews 10:25

The church is a gathering place for worship and growth. But
depending on your background and experiences, the idea of
church may conjure up mixed emotions for you. Maybe you loved
going to church as a child but haven't been back since that college
professor made you doubt the idea of faith. Maybe you come
from a church steeped in formality and tradition, and you have

memories of sitting on hard pews, in uncomfortable clothes, having to keep quiet. Perhaps someone in the church embarrassed or hurt you, and the experience turned you off in a way that has made going back difficult. Or maybe you have had positive, healthy experiences with the church and continue to go regularly but don't always feel you are getting the most out of it.

Your experience with the local church—good, bad, or indifferent—shapes your view of church attendance and membership today. Unfortunately, church has been done wrong almost as much as it has been done right through the years. It has been the source of much exclusion and pain. If you have experienced that, know it was not a reflection of God but of flawed, wrong church leaders. Church has also been the seat of hope, joy, and true community, as it should be. No matter what your early experiences or associations with the church have been, we encourage you to take a fresh look at a healthy, Bible-based church in your community. Spiritual health is the foundation of overall health and wellness, and your connection with a body of like-minded believers is an important part of that foundation.

Studies now confirm what believers have known for a long time: church makes you healthier in every way.

True connection with a strong, local church is critical for your spiritual growth and for your physical, emotional, and mental well-being. Studies now confirm what believers have known for a long time: church makes you healthier in every way. In addition to the spiritual growth benefits detailed below, regular church attendance also boosts immunity, decreases blood pressure, increases contentment, and can add as many as three years to your life.[1]

The church is a family. When you became a Christian—whether that was fifteen minutes ago or fifteen years ago—you became part of God's universal family. In every corner of the world, God's universal family meets together in smaller, local gatherings to worship and learn about God and to find community with one another. Being a member of a local church family is part of God's process for developing you into the new you. It is part of his process for growing you.

Sometimes the idea of becoming a church member can be a little intimidating. But really, the concept of membership is everywhere in our culture. You become a member at the gym or at the local wholesale club. You go to the drugstore, opt into its membership program, and walk out with a little discount card on your keychain. You sign up for a book club or the PTA, and consider yourself an active member alongside other like-minded people. Becoming a member of something is a familiar concept.

Interestingly, this idea of people coming together for membership in a common group was something the apostle Paul wrote about in one of his letters to early Christians. In fact, many believe the term *member* originated from his writing. Paul reached into the medical world and borrowed the concept that the body is made up of many types of members. Hands, arms, eyes, and feet are all different parts, yet all these parts and more come together to form a singular body. He applied the analogy to the Christian world to show that, as believers, we are all members of one body, one family.

> But our bodies have many parts, and God has put each part just where he wants it. How strange a body would be if it had only one part! Yes, there are many parts, but only one body. The eye can never say to the hand, "I don't need you." The head can't say to the feet, "I don't need you." . . . All of you together are Christ's body, and each of you is a part of it. (1 Cor. 12:18–21, 27)

Just as your head, hands, eyes, and feet are all needed to make your body function properly, all the parts of God's family are needed to form his church. In turn, the church helps you to continue growing in spiritual health by providing these main things:

94

- a place to build healthy relationships
- a place to use your gifts
- a place to grow
- a place to belong to something bigger than yourself

Let's look at each one in more detail.

A Place to Build Healthy Relationships

You weren't created to be alone. You need good people in your life. But once you are out of school and into the rhythm of adulthood, finding the kind of healthy relationships you know you need is often difficult. The limits of your social circle become your family members, coworkers, and maybe a few parents from your kids' sports teams. While these relationships are great, they are generally relationships of convenience. You also need intentional friendships with others who are on the same faith journey you are on—those who are getting to know God more deeply every day, who can come alongside you and be there for you through the ups and downs of life. Consider this truth:

> Two people are better off than one, for they can help each other succeed. If one person falls, the other can reach out and help. But someone who falls alone is in real trouble. Likewise, two people lying close together can keep each other warm. But how can one be warm alone? A person standing alone can be attacked and defeated, but two can stand back-to-back and conquer. Three are even better, for a triple-braided cord is not easily broken. (Eccles. 4:9–12)

In the local church, you can find people who are on a similar path, people you can turn to and confide in when you have doubts and questions, people who will cry with you when things are hard and share your joy in the good times. These types of intentional relationships are essential to your spiritual health (not to mention your physical, emotional, and mental health), as we will discuss much more in the next chapter.

A Place to Use Your Gifts

You were born with unique gifts and talents; you need a place to make sure those gifts and talents are being put to their highest and best use. The local church provides an environment in which you can use your gifts and talents for the benefit of God and others. This is part of God's plan for you to experience significance. Paul couldn't have been much more straightforward about this when writing to his friend Timothy: "Do not neglect the gift that is in you" (1 Tim. 4:14 NKJV).

> *When you use your gifts and talents in accordance with what God is doing around you, incredible things will happen.*

When you use your gifts and talents in accordance with what God is doing around you, incredible things will happen. You will feel alive and connected to a greater purpose. You will feel the power of God in your life as you do what you are good at to serve him. You will be a help and encouragement to the people around you.

Whether you are a musician, a tech person, someone who enjoys working with kids, a leader of people, or someone with a personality perfect for welcoming others, you can play a specific role suited to your gifts in your local church. You may know exactly how you are gifted. If so, getting plugged in should be easy for you. If you are unsure about how to serve, many spiritual gift assessments can help you figure out how you are wired. You can find one at NewYouBook.com. Or ask a leader in your church what type of assessments your church has available. (More on this in chapter 12.)

A Place to Grow

Being part of a church gives you the perfect opportunity to grow. Simply getting together with other believers, singing songs of worship, and hearing the Bible being taught in an applicable way will help you grow spiritually. Plus, when you are involved in a good church, you will learn about the personal disciplines you need to exercise to grow—disciplines such as praying and reading the Bible on your own, worshiping God in everyday moments, and forming deep relationships with other believers outside the church service. (For more on the disciplines of a growing faith, go to NewYouBook.com.)

If you aren't moving toward God, you are falling away. There is no such thing as spiritual stagnation. Taking steps of growth in a strong, local church will keep you moving in the direction of spiritual health rather than drifting toward a life of less than.

A Place to Belong to Something Bigger than Yourself

Whenever I (Nelson) watch a football game—which isn't that often, to be honest—I can't help but get fixated on those guys in the stands. You know the ones. They are usually shirtless with full body paint, face paint, and crazy glasses or hats. They put the original meaning ("fanatic") back in the term *fan*. Most of us who root for our favorite sports teams usually do so to a lesser degree, but we really aren't so different from our friends who take fandom to the next level. We are all acting out of something intrinsic to our nature.

The passion we feel for our favorite sports teams is one small indication that we are wired to belong to something bigger than ourselves. We all have a desire to be part of something that matters. I want to make a difference with my life. You want to make a difference with your life. We all want to be part of something great, something that transforms a city, something that makes people's lives better. But there is only so much we can do on our own. When we choose to connect with something bigger, like the church, we can have incredible impact.

A friend once told me, "If you want to do something that matters, figure out where God is working and link up with him in that work." Being an active part of a local church allows you to do exactly that. God is constantly at work in his church. As you see what he is doing, and choose to connect with him in it, you can become part of something much bigger than yourself—something that influences lives for the better in the here and now and for eternity.

God created the church so that you would have a place to engage, to worship, to learn, and to grow. A major part of taking responsibility for your spiritual health is connecting with a church if you aren't already or connecting more deeply if you are. Dig in. Be open to relationships with others. Put your gifts to use. Commit to a daily time with God during the week so that you go to church prepared to hear from him. Look for how God is working through your church and join him. As you do these things, God will meet you in them. He will grow you. You will be even closer to being the new you that you want to be.

Small Steps to the New You

1. Seek out a healthy, Bible-based church in your area.

2. Commit to being in church every weekend, as much as possible.

3. Take one step toward deeper engagement with your church.

11

finding good friends

The Health Benefits of Doing Life with Others

Friendship is born at that moment when one person says to another, "What! You too? I thought I was the only one."

C. S. Lewis

This is my commandment: Love each other in the same way I have loved you. There is no greater love than to lay down one's life for one's friends.

John 15:12–13

The quality of your life is determined by the quality of your relationships. That sentence is worth repeating. *The quality of your life is determined by the quality of your relationships.* Do you believe that is true? Do you live as if it is true? Do you invest deeply in healthy relationships? Or do you skim the surface? Do you allow yourself to be fully known? Or do you hide? Do you take the initiative to make plans with friends and family? Or are you more of a loner? Your approach to relationships will largely direct the course of your life.

God designed it this way. He created us with a need to be in relationship with others. That is why a lack of good relationships leaves us with a terrible feeling—loneliness. Loneliness is a danger sign. It is the body's way of telling us that if we don't connect with others soon, we are going to be in trouble. It is a warning flag telling us that something important is missing.

As we dig further into this idea of complete health in Christ, built on the foundation of spiritual health, you need to understand the connection between the quality of the relationships you have and the quality of your health. Studies show that loneliness, if left unchecked, can cause some significant physical, mental, and emotional health problems. Loneliness raises the levels of stress hormones and inflammation in the body, which increases the risk of heart disease, arthritis, type 2 diabetes, and many other ailments. People who are lonely often overeat, drink to excess, exercise less, and suffer from higher incidents of depression. They also suffer from much higher rates of suicide.[1]

Your approach to relationships will largely direct the course of your life.

Loneliness has been linked to cognitive decline and is now thought to be a predictable precursor to dementia and Alzheimer's disease. A recent study that examined eight thousand participants every two years for a twelve-year period found that those who struggled with increasing feelings of loneliness had the highest instances of cognitive decline. On average, these people experienced a rate of decline that was 20 percent faster than that of people who did not feel lonely or isolated.[2]

None of this should be surprising. God spelled it out for us in the first book of the Bible. After creating the earth, the animals, and the first human being, God said, "It is not good for the man to be alone" (Gen. 2:18). So he made a companion for the man, creating the first human relationship. And throughout Scripture, God gives us his insight into how to nurture and grow quality human relationships. Quality is key.

The interesting thing about loneliness is that it is a subjective emotion. It doesn't have much to do with the number of relationships in your life but with the quality of those relationships. Loneliness isn't based on whether you live alone or have family close by. Marriage isn't the cure, and neither is children. Loneliness is determined by whether or not you feel alone. You can feel alone in a marriage if your marriage isn't supportive. And you can feel supported and loved while living alone if you have a network of healthy relationships. As one study of this phenomenon concluded, "People can be socially isolated and not feel lonely; they simply prefer a more hermitic existence. Likewise, people can feel lonely even when surrounded by lots of people, especially if the relationships are not emotionally rewarding."[3]

Let us repeat once more: the quality of your life will be determined by the quality of your relationships. And now we could add that the quality of your health will be largely determined by the quality of your relationships. Undeniably, developing good, fulfilling relationships is crucial to your overall well-being. So how can you get started? By developing the habit of friendship.

The Habit of Friendship

Healthy, supportive relationships don't happen by accident. They take intentionality. They take a decision to practice the habit of friendship. Being proactive in your friendships makes a world of difference in the quality of your connections with other people. The effort is definitely worth the reward. Here are some ways to practice the habit of friendship:

- make friends by being a friend first
- choose to enjoy life with your friends
- support your friends in both good times and bad
- take the risk of making new connections

Let's take a look at each one in more detail.

Make Friends by Being a Friend First

You have to be a friend to have a friend. Have you heard that little piece of advice before? It couldn't be truer. Most of us spend a great deal of time and energy looking for people who will listen to us, accept us, share our point of view, be there for us when we need them . . . and yet we spend little energy thinking about how we can do these things for other people. We have to be a friend first by being intentional about offering friendship to others. The apostle John put it this way: "Dear children, let's not merely say that we love each other; let us show the truth by our actions" (1 John 3:18).

Your actions toward the people in your life will show whether you are truly being a friend or whether you are just on the lookout for someone who will be a friend to you. Ask yourself these questions:

- Am I respectful of other opinions and points of view?
- Am I quick to apologize when I say or do something wrong?
- Do I forgive easily when a friend has offended me?
- Do I listen well and respond thoughtfully?
- Am I available when a friend needs me, even if it is inconvenient?
- Do I give my time and energy willingly?

Talk is cheap, as they say. Saying you are someone's friend doesn't require much sacrifice—but being a good friend does.

Being a friend is an intentional choice to love, day by day. In the words of Jesus: "This is my commandment: Love each other in the same way I have loved you. There is no greater love than to lay down one's life for one's friends" (John 15:12–13).

Choose to Enjoy Life with Your Friends

We know you are busy. Between work, family, and other obligations, you probably have a hard time squeezing anything else in. Unfortunately, when life is hectic, time spent hanging out with friends is the first thing to go—but it shouldn't be. To create and maintain healthy relationships, you have to be intentional about scheduling time to enjoy life with your friends. Take the time to grab lunch or dinner, see a movie, or go for a walk in a nearby park. Catch up with each other. Relax. Laugh.

Hard work is a given. There are bills to pay and mouths to feed. But you get to choose how much fun you have. You get to choose how you balance work and play. Much of your happiness is a result of the time you allow yourself to spend enjoying life, especially with other people. You need to be able to break away from the stress of the everyday and make time to enjoy being with friends.

Time is the heartbeat of every strong friendship. Without it, distance slips in, effort begins to dip, and friendships that were once strong start to dry up. Not only is this bad for the relationship in question but it is also bad for your physical, mental, and emotional health. The best way around the problem is to begin putting time with friends on your calendar, just as you would a work meeting or a school event. Simply writing down when you are going to see your friends will help you make a subtle mental shift to seeing that time as nonnegotiable.

You have to be intentional about spending time enjoying life with the people who matter to you.

Friendships flourish through shared experience and by spending unstructured time together. Neither of these things will happen by default. You have to be intentional about spending time enjoying life with the people who matter to you.

Support Your Friends in Both Good Times and Bad

Do you have people in your life who encourage you to be your best? Do you have friends who are there for you when life is hard? Do you support other people when they need you and share in their happiness when things are going well? Studies show that, despite our overly connected world, the number of true confidants people have has been steadily dropping over the last few decades.[4] While we may have many friends on social media or many casual acquaintances, we aren't living life with our friends as well as generations past.

You need to have people you can really talk to and be yourself with no matter what is going on, and your friends need you to be there when things are happening in their lives. Paul put it this way: "When we get together, I want to encourage you in your faith, but I also want to be encouraged by yours" (Rom. 1:12).

A certain phrase is often used in Christian circles: do life together. Doing life together is exactly what it sounds like—finding a group of friends you can walk with through life's ups and downs, friends you can encourage and be encouraged by. These are friends you can call on a Friday night to go grab pizza with. These are friends you feel comfortable having over, even if there is a pile of laundry on the couch and you are in the same T-shirt you slept in. When something is wrong, they are there for you and vice versa. There is no pretense, simply a mutual desire to be and have the type of friends we all need.

We all want to be known. We don't want to have to perform and make good impressions in our friendships. We want to be able to be ourselves and to be accepted for who we are. Again, developing the kinds of relationships in which this can happen takes intentionality. Sometimes it takes stepping outside of your comfort zone and taking a risk. But the reward is sweet.

Take the Risk of Making New Connections

Take a step back for a minute and think about the friendships in your life. Can you say that you have the types of friendships we have been discussing? Do you have friends with whom you would feel comfortable developing a deeper, more meaningful, more trusting relationship? Most people don't. Most people feel the void of these kinds of connected, growing, encouraging friendships.

In the last chapter, we talked about why it is so important to get connected to a healthy, local church. Your need for strong relationships is one more reason. Most churches offer small groups—and small groups are the best way to begin growing friendships with like-minded people who are also looking for a few good friends to do life with. If you aren't familiar with the concept, a small group is simply a group of ten to fifteen people who get together on a regular basis to learn more about God, create connections, and have some fun.

Getting into a small group is not a guarantee that you will suddenly have great relationships. But you will find yourself surrounded by people who care about you, people who are on a similar life path, people you can be yourself around. You will find people you enjoy hanging out with. You will learn to carry their burdens, and they will be willing to carry yours. You will have the opportunity to encourage them and receive encouragement from them when you need it. And through your small group, or maybe through a series of small groups (depending on how your church is set up), you will begin to identify the people

> *There is no better place to find others who will help you grow than in a church, among people who are all seeking after God and his best.*

105

you want to go even deeper with. You will find those friends you will look at a few years from now and wonder how you ever got along without them.

There is nothing wrong with being intentional about the places you choose to find friends. In fact, there is a lot right with it. And there is no better place to find others who will help you grow than in a church, among people who are all seeking after God and his best. Your health depends on it.

A Word to Introverts

I (Jennifer) know how intimidating stepping out of your comfort zone and joining a small group of strangers can be. I understand the hesitation, because I am one of you. I am much more comfortable on my own than in a room full of people, especially people I don't know well. If you know joining a small group is important but are reticent, I have been where you are. But now that I am on the other side of countless successful small groups (and a few unsuccessful ones—it is part of the process), I couldn't be happier I took the plunge into intentional community.

When my husband, Brian, and I moved to New York City in our midtwenties, we didn't know anyone. We were in a new place with no connections. After a few months, we found a great, healthy church, but we still didn't have any friends we felt a deep bond with. When our church started promoting small groups, I was torn. I knew we needed to join a group, but I didn't want to join a group. My husband is a classic extrovert, so he was excited and ready to get involved. I decided to do what I knew was right, even if it made me uncomfortable. And I can't tell you how glad I am that I did.

I joined a women's group and went to those first few meetings with butterflies in my stomach. I probably didn't say much. But soon the relationships began to influence me. I was surrounded by people I could relate to. I began to make friends. Another woman in the group and I went on to colead a group of our own a few months later. Then in the next few years, Brian and I were part of countless couples' groups together.

Now, well over a decade later, the greatest friends in our lives are people we initially met through a small group. They are the people we have gone through so much life with—job changes, promotions, marital challenges, deaths in the family, births. We have laughed until it hurt together, cried together, vacationed together, grown in our relationships with God together. I don't know what I would have done without them. Did we bond with everyone we were in a group with? Of course not; that is not even the goal. But groups helped us identify the people who became our people. And they helped us grow deeper in our walk with Jesus, alongside others on a similar journey. The same can be true for you.

An old cliché says, "Life begins at the end of your comfort zone." It couldn't be truer. Even though you may be anxious, even though you may be uncomfortable, I can't encourage you enough to take the step of getting involved in a small group through your local church. You need intentional, healthy relationships for your own well-being as much as everyone you meet needs them for theirs. We are all in this together.

Taking the Risk

The quality of your life is determined by the quality of your relationships. A lack of healthy relationships in your life can cause significant physical, mental, and emotional problems. Friendships with other believers will grow and challenge you spiritually. They will increase your spiritual health, the foundation of your overall health and wellness. The evidence is undeniable. There is no good reason for you not to be intentional about creating healthier friendships—and every reason to do so. God can't force you to make choices to develop the type of friendships that will produce spiritual growth. Once again, the choice is yours.

Is it time for you to take a risk? Is it time for you to step out of your comfort zone? You can do it. As you take this journey toward complete health, make quality relationships part of it. What you gain will be more than worth what you have to venture.

Small Steps to the New You

1. Make a list of the supportive friends in your life. How many do you have? How authentic are these relationships?

2. Seek out information about small groups at your church.

3. Sign up for a small group and go!

12

the power of serving

Seven Ways to Change the World

It is one of the most beautiful compensations of life, that no man can sincerely try to help another without helping himself.

Ralph Waldo Emerson

Those who refresh others will themselves be refreshed.

Proverbs 11:25

I (Nelson) don't usually read *Forbes* magazine, but I can't keep myself from picking up the yearly edition in which the magazine announces its roll of billionaires. I like to check whether or not I made the list. I know this may surprise you, but I have never seen my name alongside Bill Gates and Warren Buffet. Before I became a Christian, I used to think making the *Forbes* list would be the ultimate sign of greatness. But God defines success differently, doesn't he? Just because the people on that list are great in the world's eyes doesn't mean they are great in God's. Then again, they may be, but if they are, it has nothing to do with their financial achievements.

The good news is that you and I don't have to be on that *Forbes* list, or any other list, to be great. God has another way for you to be great. And God's path to greatness is also something that is a key to your health. Isn't it just like God to arrange things that way? You can wake up every morning and be extraordinary. You can go to bed every night knowing you are partnering with God to make a difference. How? By being willing to help others. Jesus said, "The greatest among you must be a servant" (Matt. 23:11).

Serving others is good for your spiritual, physical, mental, and emotional well-being. Though helping others may not get you featured in a magazine, doing so in ways both big and small will have a significant effect on the quality of your life and your overall health. In fact, a principle—often referred to as the Greatness Principle—says that when you bless others, God blesses you. (Pick up our book *The Greatness Principle: Finding Significance and Joy by Serving Others* to learn more.)

Of course, many benefits of serving others are tied to the benefits of having strong relationships in your life (chapter 11), since serving often leads to deep connection with the ones you are serving or the ones you are serving alongside. Serving is also scientifically linked to a longer life-span, better pain management, lower blood pressure, and greater happiness.

Studies show that when you do something to help someone else, the reward center of your brain pumps out the mood-elevating neurotransmitter dopamine, creating what researchers call a "helper's high."[1] That sense of well-being has long-range effects.

How to Start Serving Others

The best way to get started serving others is simply to become aware of the needs around you. You come in contact with countless needs and chances to help others day in and day out, but you won't see them until you make an effort to become aware that they exist. Much like you notice pregnant women when you are pregnant and blue cars when you buy one, you will start seeing opportunities to serve you never would have noticed before when helping others becomes something you actively think about.

Here are seven ways to start seeing and meeting needs around you, doing your health and well-being a favor in the process.

Encourage the People around You

Encouraging someone with your words is one of the simplest yet most powerful ways you can help. As Paul wrote, "Don't use foul or abusive language. Let everything you say be good and helpful, so that your words will be an encouragement to those who hear them" (Eph. 4:29).

Here are a few practical ways you can use your words to encourage those around you:

- pay your coworker a sincere compliment
- congratulate your child on a job well done
- listen to a friend who needs to talk and respond thoughtfully
- intentionally build up your spouse

Help Someone in Need

When you see a need, don't ignore it. Be willing to inconvenience yourself in order to help someone who needs help. As a friend of mine says, "Small things done with great love will change the world."

Helping others is contagious. By being quick to lend a hand to someone in need, you could spark a revolution. When someone sees you offering help, they are likely to do the same when given the opportunity.

"Small things done with great love will change the world."

111

Imagine the difference we could make if we all decided to help another person every day. Here are a few practical ways you can help the people around you:

- carry an elderly person's groceries to their car
- help a mom lift her stroller up a flight of stairs
- take a meal to a family who is going through a hard time
- offer to babysit for free for a friend who has young children

Invite Your Friends to Church

Inviting your friends who don't know Jesus to church is a great act of service. I know inviting them to a ball game or out to dinner is easier than inviting them to church, but push through the intimidation and take that step of faith.

Here is some news that might make things a little easier: statistics show that you are actually risking very little when you invite your friends to church. Around 50 percent of your unchurched friends will go with you the first time you ask. That percentage goes up substantially with a second or third invitation.[2] Believe me, you will not offend any of your friends by inviting them to church. Even if they say no, they will be touched that you cared enough to ask. And just think of what could happen if they say yes. Here is more from Paul: "Live wisely among those who are not believers, and make the most of every opportunity" (Col. 4:5).

When you invite your friends to church, you are inviting them to a place where they can learn about their Creator and have their deepest needs met, where they can find friends who will support and encourage them, where they can learn what it means to follow Jesus, where they can begin to take responsibility for their own spiritual health.

As Andy Stanley says, "Following Jesus will make your life better and make you better at life."[3] What better way could there be to bless your friends than to invite them into that opportunity?

And if following Jesus is something you are still exploring, you can bring your friends along to explore with you.

Connect with Your Family

Even though you may have the best of intentions to keep your family members at the top of your priority list, all too often they slip toward the bottom when things get busy. Be intentional about blessing your family members every chance you get.

Honoring your relationship with your family is important to God, as evidenced by these Scripture passages:

> Honor your father and mother. Then you will live a long, full life in the land the LORD your God is giving you. (Exod. 20:12)

> Husbands, love your wives, just as Christ loved the church and gave himself up for her. (Eph. 5:25 NIV)

> Do not provoke your children to anger by the way you treat them. Rather, bring them up with the discipline and instruction that comes from the Lord. (Eph. 6:4)

> But those who won't care for their relatives, especially those in their own household, have denied the true faith. (1 Tim. 5:8)

Your willingness to proactively serve your family members will create stronger family ties and be a great example to onlookers. Here are a few practical ways you can connect with your family right away:

- schedule a date night with your spouse
- spend some one-on-one time with each of your kids
- call your parents
- plan a trip to visit your extended family

Pray for Your Friends

Praying for your friends is a powerful way to help them, without them even knowing about it. Jesus's brother James wrote, "The earnest prayer of a righteous person has great power and produces wonderful results" (James 5:16).

> When you see a need in a friend's life, praying about it may be the most helpful thing you can do.

When you see a need in a friend's life, praying about it may be the most helpful thing you can do. Pray and act, but even when you can't act, always pray. Prayers truly make a difference. Here are a few ways you can start praying for your friends today:

- pray that they will be sensitive to god's guidance in their lives
- pray for their health and safety
- pray for their family relationships
- pray for your relationship with them
- pray about specific circumstances they are facing

Serve Your City or Town

Maybe you have never thought much about this, but God has you living where you are for a reason. He wants you to impact your city or town in a way only you can. Consider this Bible verse: "Work for the peace and prosperity of the city where I sent you. . . . Pray to the LORD for it, for its welfare will determine your welfare" (Jer. 29:7).

You are called to engage the area you call home. Bless your city or town by showing the people who live there the love of Jesus in action. Here are a few practical ways you can start serving your city or town:

- get involved with your church's community outreach ministries

- serve at a local homeless shelter
- serve at a pregnancy crisis center
- sign up to build houses with Habitat for Humanity
- tutor children in low-income areas
- say thank you to your local police officers and firefighters

Join a Volunteer Team at Your Church

Left to our own devices, we can be lazy about serving others. Over time, selfishness creeps in, and we forget to focus outward. This happens to all of us. Joining a volunteer team at your church is a good way to make sure that serving others regularly is a priority. Doing so will also give you the chance to use the gifts God has given you to serve him. As we discussed in chapter 10, you are wired to plug into the local church and volunteer in a specific way. If you are a gifted singer or musician, you may be perfectly positioned to meet a need on your church's worship team. If you are good with kids, maybe you can use that skill to help with the children's programs. Maybe you want to volunteer but aren't sure exactly what to do. Identify what you feel drawn to. You can also take the spiritual gifts test at NewYouBook.com or ask a leader in your church what types of assessments your church has available.

When you plug in and start serving at your church, you will

- get to know new people and begin forming healthy relationships;
- experience the excitement of putting your gifts to use;
- feel better physically;
- be happier; and
- grow spiritually.

Stay open and sensitive to God's guidance. Act on small opportunities that present themselves daily. Pay attention to your passions and gifting as you think about how you can serve in bigger, ongoing ways. When you do those things, you will be able to step forward into the world ready to serve others well—and boost your own health and happiness immeasurably at the same time. Plus, you will have the joy of knowing you are engaging with God in a meaningful, tangible way. What could be greater than that?

Small Steps to the New You

1. Choose to be aware of the needs around you.

2. Act on small opportunities that present themselves daily.

3. Pay attention to your passions and gifting and use them to serve others.

small steps
to better
emotional
health

13

managing your emotions

What Is Emotional Health and How Do You Preserve It?

I have chosen to be happy because it is good for my health.

Voltaire

But the Holy Spirit produces this kind of fruit in our lives: love, joy, peace, patience, kindness, goodness, faithfulness, gentleness, and self-control.

Galatians 5:22–23

A friend of mine (Jennifer) who was struggling with being overweight and dealing with some physical health issues confided in me that as she became unhealthier physically, she also started having some emotional difficulties. (Don't worry, I am not breaching confidence. I asked her if I could share her story anonymously, and she agreed.) She wasn't clinically depressed. Her emotional challenges weren't debilitating. Still, she knew the

119

way she was beginning to feel about herself was interfering with her day-to-day activities.

She was having a harder time bouncing back when things went wrong. She was plagued with a sense that she wasn't good enough and people didn't really like her. She began to distance herself emotionally from her husband, her kids, and her closest friends—not because she wanted to, necessarily; she just didn't feel she had what it took to engage with them well. Have you ever been there? I have.

Physical and emotional health are inextricably linked, with spiritual health being the foundation for both. It is not surprising that as obesity rates and related health problems have skyrocketed, so have rates of depression and anxiety. The two areas play on and feed into each other, so much so that the cause and effect are not clear. In fact, as depression rates rise, so do obesity rates.

As was true with my friend, when someone sees their physical health slipping away, they are at a much higher risk of becoming anxious, depressed, and isolated from those they love. As that happens, they have even less drive to take the necessary steps to regain physical health, so the problem builds on itself. They may even overeat as a coping mechanism, which leads to even greater weight gain and even more depression or anxiety. And the cycle continues. Whether poor physical health or poor emotional health is the catalyst, the two are intertwined.

Getting a Grip on Emotional Health

Emotional health isn't quite as easy to pin down as physical health. There are no numbers to measure just how emotionally fit you are. Psychologists define emotional health as an overall psychological well-being. It is a combination of the way you feel about yourself, the quality of your relationships, and your ability to manage your feelings and deal with difficulty. People who are emotionally healthy have a sense of contentment and a zest for life. They are

120

able to laugh and have fun with those around them. They rebound from adversity quickly and deal with stress well. The relationships in their lives are good, and their sense of self-esteem is strong.[1]

Even though it is more subjective than quantifiable, emotional health is a key component of your ability to be the new you that you are working toward becoming. When you aren't emotionally healthy, your body suffers as a result. The negative thoughts and feelings you experience create chemical reactions in your physiology that can lead to weakened immunity, chest pains, shortness of breath, fatigue, back pain, high blood pressure, digestion issues, and more.[2] Poor emotional health makes you less likely to dive into the healthy lifestyle changes you need to make to get your body where you want it to be. It may also keep you from wanting to engage in the disciplines that are important to your spiritual health, both corporately and privately. This isn't an issue to be taken lightly. Poor emotional health can completely derail your wellness in every other area.

While the majority of us won't deal with emotional problems that cross the line into diagnosable distress, we are all likely to experience some level of difficulty as a result of poor emotional health. Being aware of some of the most common emotional stressors and having a plan for dealing with them can help you sidestep emotional pitfalls.

Keys for Maintaining Emotional Strength

Personal, relational, and occupational issues are the stuff that emotional triggers are made of. The varieties of problems that can threaten your well-being are too numerous to list. Here are just a few of the things you may deal with at different points in your life that can cause emotional strain:

- a traumatic event
- trouble at work
- an increase in financial obligation

121

- discrimination
- competition with others
- marriage difficulties
- problems with children
- caring for an elderly family member
- issues with extended family
- physical illness or injury

Any of these, given the right combination of circumstances, has the potential to send you spiraling if you aren't careful. But you can protect yourself and your emotional health by doing these things consistently:

- sidestep surprise
- focus on the positive
- strengthen your foundation
- seek counseling

Let's look at each one in more detail.

Sidestep Surprise

The situations that have the most potential to shake you are the ones that come out of nowhere: an unexpected diagnosis, a surprising layoff, an unforeseeable accident. When a problem you weren't expecting sideswipes you, it is easy to find yourself panicked and vulnerable to a host of reactions. One of the biggest keys to maintaining your emotional equilibrium is choosing not to be surprised when problems show up.

We live in a fallen world full of tough circumstances and deep disappointments. Jesus said to expect this: "Here on earth you will have many trials and sorrows. But take heart, because I have overcome the world" (John 16:33).

When you accept the reality that problems and pain are an inevitable part of life, you won't be surprised when they come along. And you can take a great deal of comfort in Jesus's promise that he has already overcome everything you will face. You have the promise of peace. Jesus never promised that life on this side of heaven would be easy, even for those who are grounded in him; he simply promised to be with us every step of the way, no matter what comes along.

Focus on the Positive

When bad circumstances threaten to steal your joy, shift your attention to the good in your life. Celebrate what God is doing around you. Focus on what is positive rather than what is negative. There is proven power in choosing to be optimistic. The story you tell yourself about the events in your life goes a long way toward creating your experience. So when you think about the hard things you

> *There is proven power in choosing to be optimistic.*

are experiencing, be intentional about finding the positive as well. Doing so is the key not only to emotional health but also to physical health, mental health, and spiritual maturity.

Positive psychology expert Dr. Martin Seligman has much to say on this issue. In his book *Flourish: A Visionary New Understanding of Happiness and Well-being*, he says:

> People tend to spend more time thinking about what is bad in life than is helpful. Worse, this focus on negative events sets us up for anxiety and depression. One way to keep this from happening is to get better at thinking about and savoring what went well. . . . To overcome our brains' natural catastrophic bent, we need to work on and practice this skill of thinking about what went well.[3]

Seligman goes on to suggest an exercise called the What-Went-Well exercise (also known as Three Blessings), which has been scientifically proven to increase emotional well-being. We describe a version of it here, with credit to him.

> Every night for one week, write down three positive events from your day—three things that went well. These can be simple things such as "My husband picked up my favorite flowers on the way home" or more important things such as "My friend just gave birth to a healthy baby boy."
>
> Next to each positive event, write down your answer to the question Why did this event happen? For example, you might write, "My husband picked up flowers because I mentioned we needed some" or "My friend had a healthy baby because God is so good and because she took such good care of herself during her pregnancy." As Seligman notes, this exercise may seem awkward at first, but keep with it and it will get easier. Hopefully looking at the positive will become a habit. Countless studies prove that as you do this exercise regularly, you will be less anxious, less depressed, and quantifiably healthier.[4]

A sense of gratitude is an important precursor to an ability to focus on the positive. Learn to say thank you for the good in your life. If you simply start looking, you will find so many things to be thankful for. Think about these things. Talk about these things. Refuse to complain. Let your subconscious hear your grateful words so it can, in turn, pull up more opportunities for gratefulness in your life. (For more on developing an attitude of gratefulness, see our book *Tongue Pierced: How the Words You Speak Transform the Life You Live.*)

Strengthen Your Foundation

There are two main categories to consider when strengthening your foundation: public activities and private disciplines. When you are feeling emotionally drained, anxious, or depressed, lean even harder on both. Make sure to be intentional about the following:

- *Your connection with your church.* Stay connected to your church, even when you may not feel like it. Get up, get dressed, and get there, no matter how hard it is. The enemy would love nothing more than to separate you from God's family when you are struggling. And on that note . . .

- *Your connection with your small group.* Don't let feelings of anxiety, depression, low self-esteem, or even just general malaise keep you from getting together with your like-minded friends. The healthy relationships in your life are critical when you are feeling emotionally drained or distraught. Let people surround you, encourage you, and help you walk through whatever is bothering you.

- *Your daily time with God.* Part of staying emotionally healthy is carving out time to get quiet with God every day. Tell him when you feel anxious. Talk to him about what you are struggling with. Read his Word and listen to how he wants to guide you. He will calm your emotions and encourage you in the right direction every time.

As you do these things on an ongoing basis, you will naturally be more prepared to deal with the difficult emotions you face day to day. When particularly emotional circumstances come up, press even harder into the One who gives you everything you need to face them with strength.

Seek Counseling

Never be ashamed to seek Christian counseling. Talking to a professional about the things going on in your life can help you process and deal with your emotions in a healthy way. And there is absolutely nothing wrong with doing so. In fact, there are many benefits.

Several years ago, before my son was born, Kelley and I (Nelson) went through a rough patch in our marriage. We had been married for a while and thought we weren't able to have children. Dealing with that reality wore on us. We began to pull away from each other emotionally. Knowing we needed some outside help, we decided to find a good marriage counselor.

At first, I was hesitant. The idea of walking into an office and talking to a stranger about the details of my marriage made me want to run in the opposite direction. Thankfully, I pushed through my doubts and chose to engage. Even though some of the sessions were difficult, I can honestly say the entire process was extremely healthy. To this day, our marriage is benefiting from what we learned.

Our experience with the marriage counselor made me appreciate the value of Christian counseling, so much so that I made a personal decision to see a counselor regularly whether I thought I needed to or not. I have discovered great benefit in the process. I expect you will too, if you decide to give it a try. As I have found, talking to a trained counselor will help you deal with emotions you didn't even realize you were having. Over time, the process will raise your emotional health quotient higher and higher and serve as a safety net to make sure nothing sends you spiraling in the other direction.

On Guard

Keeping yourself emotionally healthy is an important step in improving your overall health and well-being. Be on the lookout for the things that can take you down the path to anxiety, panic, or depression. When you see these things threatening your well-being, take intentional action to counter them. Do everything in your power to guard against the attacks being levied at your heart and mind from every angle, even as you trust God to do his part to protect you. As you recognize and take responsibility for the state of your emotional health, your physical, mental, and spiritual health will also benefit—and you will be well on your way to becoming the new you.

Small Steps to the New You

1. Do the What-Went-Well exercise before you go to bed tonight. Commit to doing it for at least one week.

2. When you feel tempted to complain, find something positive to say instead.

3. Have lunch or dinner with a friend from your small group and ask them about the good things going on in their life.

4. Find a Christian counselor in your area and establish a relationship.

14

energy in motion

Practices for Increasing Your Productivity,
Resilience, Focus, and Endurance

Performance, health and happiness are grounded in the skillful
management of energy.

Jim Loehr

But those who trust in the LORD will find new strength.
They will soar high on wings like eagles.
They will run and not grow weary.
They will walk and not faint.

Isaiah 40:31

I (Nelson) have a colleague in New York who loves to run the New
York City Marathon. Each year he spends months training for
that November day when he gets up before dawn to run twenty-six
miles. One of his goals is to keep a consistent pace throughout.
He doesn't want to run a few miles, then walk a few miles, then

run again, then walk the last five, like so many marathoners do. He likes the challenge of trying to maintain the same speed the entire race. "Life is a marathon," he has told me on more than one occasion. "Doing this helps me push through every day of my regular life without slowing down." While I respect my friend, I completely disagree with his outlook.

Life Is Not a Marathon

Life is not a marathon, and it shouldn't be looked at as one. Life is better viewed as a series of short sprints with periods of rest in between. Think about the way most professional athletes train. They expend a huge amount of energy for a season, and then they have the off-season to rest and recover. They repeat that cycle over and over for as long as they play their game. If they tried to forge ahead without the rest period, they wouldn't have very long careers.

These high-level athletes know and apply a principle that most people never think much about. We like to call it the stress-and-release cycle. Our bodies, minds, and emotions all work best when we stretch (or stress) them for a period of time and then release the pressure. When we push ourselves for a while and then allow ourselves to take a break, we have the chance to recover. That recovery period is when growth happens. Our bodies' systems go to work integrating everything we experienced and learned during the push period (childbirth would be a great analogy here, but we will spare the male readers), making us more prepared for the next go-around. But when we treat life like a marathon, we never get the opportunity to recharge. Instead, we slowly become run down because we aren't operating within the structure of how we function best.

God is the one behind this concept. He put it into practice when he created the world. He worked diligently for six days and

129

then rested for a day. We are designed to do the same—to work, then rest; to sprint, then recover. When we approach life this way, we are more resilient, have more clarity, and have an easier time controlling our energy in a positive way.

You probably know something about time management, but maybe you have never thought about the idea of energy management. Managing your energy well is just as important, if not more important, as managing your time well. More energy equals more productivity. More energy means more resilience so you can get back up again when something knocks you down. More energy means having more of your best to give to the people around you, having more enthusiasm to engage with God's purposes, and being able to finish each day feeling good.

On the flip side, low energy has dangerous effects for every area of our well-being—but that is where most of us live. We walk around half human, half zombie, in search of our next cup of coffee or a few minutes of rest. Living on low energy means we handle the situations in our lives less effectively and with less grace than we'd like. It means we don't have the stamina to do the things that are good for us, such as practicing disciplines that lead to health. Low energy makes us irritable and less fun to be around. It puts us in the mind-set of counting the minutes until bedtime instead of making the minutes count. Can you relate?

Energy Equations

The Latin derivative for the word *emotion* literally means "energy in motion." So emotion equals energy in motion. That is why discovering how to manage your energy well will give you the emotional (and physical) get-up-and-go it takes to become the new you. When you have more energy, you will approach life more proactively. You will want to get out and move your body. You will put more emphasis on getting good rest so you don't lose your enthusiasm. You will be able to invest happily in activities and relationships that may have seemed like a chore to you before. More energy equals more productivity, resilience, focus, and endurance.

The way to manage your energy over the long haul is to begin viewing your life as a series of short sprints with recovery periods in between. Here are some simple tips for maximizing your energy that you can layer

> *More energy equals more productivity, resilience, focus, and endurance.*

on top of that foundation. Some of these points are covered at length in other chapters, so we will just mention them briefly here.

More Alignment = More Energy

When you are walking in the center of what God has planned for you, you experience excitement and peace that go beyond understanding. That sense of alignment produces energy. The opposite is also true: misalignment leads to low energy. Take time to align yourself with the calling God has placed on your life each and every day. And note the inherent effect here: as more alignment gives you more energy, that energy in turn helps you engage in the daily practices that lead to more alignment—practices such as morning devotions, focused prayer time, and serving others.

More Cooperation = More Energy

God created you with certain rhythms and tendencies that are unique to your makeup. Paying attention to what those are and learning to cooperate with them will help you have more energy every day. For example, you are likely either a morning person or a night owl. Whichever way you have been wired, work with it; don't fight against it. In the same way, you naturally go through energy peaks and valleys throughout the day that are different from those of the people around you. Recognize when the peaks are for you and plan your highest-energy tasks during those times.

The alternative only leads to frustration. Figure out what works best for the way you have been designed and then operate within those boundaries.

More Awareness = More Energy

This one works in conjunction with the previous one. Thanks to the way God wired you, certain activities energize you and others drain you. These are different for everyone. For example, I (Nelson) am not good at counseling people. It absolutely zaps me. But a guy I work with loves counseling others; he walks out of counseling sessions energized. God created the two of us very differently in that area, and we are happiest and most effective when we work in light of that reality.

Take time to align yourself with the calling God has placed on your life each and every day.

To have more energy, become aware of the things that fill you up and do those things. Look at your to-do list from yesterday and put a plus sign next to the items that energized you and a minus sign next to the ones that drained you. With intentional awareness over time, you can learn to focus on what you are wired for and shift away from what you aren't.

A Regular Rest Day = More Energy

Your rest day, or your Sabbath, is your recovery period after the sprint of a busy week. This is simply a twenty-four-hour period when you unplug and spend time focusing on your family and on God. For one full day, you relinquish control of the universe back to its rightful owner. Choosing to step away from your business-as-usual schedule, no matter how busy you are or what is going on, proves your trust in God's control. You need to take a rest day for your own well-being. If you don't, you will begin to feel the wear on your body, your spirit, your mind, and your emotions pretty quickly. A day of rest renews your energy, your

132

focus, and your commitment to keep doing all that God has called you to do.

Regular Exercise = More Energy

As we have already discussed, walking is one of the best forms of exercise. And it just so happens that walking will give you an incredible boost of energy. Every minute you spend walking will be returned to you in productivity later in the day. To read more about the benefits of regular walking and other exercise, turn back to chapter 8.

More Hydration = More Energy

Again, staying well hydrated keeps the energy level in your body where it should be. The amount of water you take in needs to match or exceed the amount of water you lose in a day—which is more than you think. Even mild dehydration can zap your energy level, your mood, and your ability to think clearly. For a refresher on the importance of drinking enough water, turn back to chapter 7.

More Health = More Energy

Of course, being physically, spiritually, emotionally, and mentally healthy will increase your energy. But for this specific point, we are referring to avoiding the common illnesses constantly floating around us. Have you ever put a kid in preschool only to have said kid pick up every illness going around and pass it along to the rest of the family? When each of my (Jennifer's) two girls started preschool, they became sick with everything imaginable . . . and they weren't stingy about sharing with Brian and me. But over time, as their immune systems strengthened, they stopped contracting everything that walked through the doors of their school. While getting sick is sometimes unavoidable, you can take certain steps to keep your immunity up and ward off those pesky germs. The following steps will look familiar:

- get enough sleep
- stay hydrated
- eat well
- exercise regularly

Plus one more big one: wash your hands. Washing your hands often with soap and warm water is the single best way you can keep yourself from getting sick. Wash long enough to sing "Happy Birthday" or the ABC song under your breath twice.

Less Weight = More Energy

Obviously, the heavier you are, the harder your body has to work to get through the day. Losing just 10 percent of your body weight can result in a significant increase in energy. Did you need another reason to shed those pounds?

Less Clutter = More Energy

Not only is clutter a distraction but it can also become an emotional stumbling block and drain your energy. A recent study asked participants to perform a task in a neatly organized room and a highly disorganized room. Across the board, the participants were less successful in the cluttered room. Not surprising, is it? A home or an office that is clean and organized rather than in chaos makes us feel better. Clutter makes us feel as if things are out of control, which is emotionally and mentally draining. To have more energy, have enough self-control to keep clutter at bay.

More Praise = More Energy

Focusing on the goodness of God will always renew your energy. Take David's words to heart: "I will praise the LORD at all times. I will constantly speak his praises" (Ps. 34:1). Let praise be the golden thread weaving through every activity of your day. This simple practice will bring you into better alignment with God, draw you deeper into his presence, and create enthusiasm in all you do. When you choose to focus your attention on the source of all the good things in your life, your energy tank will be continually refilled.

Small Steps to the New You

1. Look over yesterday's to-do list. Put a plus sign next to every activity that filled you with energy and a minus sign next to what drained you. Going forward, try to focus more of your attention on the things that are a plus.

2. Take fifteen minutes to declutter and organize your desk or one room in your home. If you think you can't finish in fifteen minutes, start anyway—and then do fifteen more minutes tomorrow.

3. Put on some praise music and sing along while you make breakfast or run errands.

15

defeating the
deadliest emotion

The Necessity of Rooting Out Bitterness

As we pour out our bitterness, God pours in his peace.

F. B. Meyer

Look after each other so that none of you fails to receive the grace
of God. Watch out that no poisonous root of bitterness grows up
to trouble you, corrupting many.

Hebrews 12:15

et's begin with a shout-out to all you beautiful people who are
blessed with a green thumb. I (Jennifer) am not. If I am being
honest, I hate gardening and yard work. I will admit it. While I
want my lawn to look nice, keeping up with it is just not one of
my favorite things, as Julie Andrews would say. Since I don't get

any pleasure or relaxation from tilling, planting, and the like, whenever I do these things, I always end up feeling I should be doing something else. Then I end up frustrated that not only am I doing a job I really don't want to be doing but I am also taking time away from other things that are much more in my lane (but that is another topic for another day). The thing I hate the most is pulling weeds.

Weeds are the worst. No matter how often you pull them, more always spring up, trying to choke the life out of everything around them. If left unchecked, they will devour any healthy growth close by. A thoughtful gardener—one much better than me—painstakingly pulls the weeds out by their roots, one by one, to make sure they don't have the opportunity to sabotage the good plants.

Even though I do not enjoy weeding, I do recognize how important it is—and how similar it is to the work we need to do to keep our emotional lives healthy. If we aren't careful, weeds will begin growing inside us. And just like the weeds in a garden, they will work to choke out the beauty around them. They can destroy our relationships, our emotional well-being, our intimacy with God, and even our physical health. Bitterness and unforgiveness in particular are deadly weeds. In fact, unaddressed bitterness is one of the greatest health risks we face.

> *Unaddressed bitterness is one of the greatest health risks we face.*

You may be thinking to yourself, *I can skip this part. I'm not bitter. Unforgiveness isn't a big problem for me.* Hopefully, you are right—but you would be a huge exception. You likely have small weeds of bitterness sprouting in your heart that you don't even recognize. Take this little litmus test: How do you feel when you hear that someone has made an unfair comment about you behind your back? What about when a family member or a coworker doesn't do something they said they would do? Or when a friend hurts your feelings? Do those things just roll off your back? You may say they do, but deep down they hurt. To pretend otherwise would be to deny the reality of your humanity.

While in seminary, I (Nelson) became friends with an older pastor who had been in ministry for many years. I was young and on fire for God. I was completely naïve about the problems pastors face during long years of ministry. While I respected this mentor of mine and learned a great deal from him, he also became a cautionary tale to me. Over the years, he had grown into a negative, bitter man. He couldn't see the bitterness in himself, but it was clear to me. I remember praying, "God, help me stay positive and passionate for you. Don't let me grow bitter." At the time, I didn't realize how powerful bitterness could be.

Over the last thirty years, I have learned just how easily these weeds can spring up and take root in an unexamined heart. At one point, I found myself heading down a similar path as my mentor. I could feel unforgiveness and bitterness getting comfortable within me. I could sense small changes in my attitude that I knew weren't healthy or Christlike. Thankfully, through a lot of prayer and through a key friendship with Steve Reynolds (author of the excellent *Bod4God* book), God showed me how to turn my heart back toward grace and forgiveness.

Bitterness is a troublemaker that creates curmudgeonly, unhappy people. The Bible goes so far as to call bitterness a root (Heb. 12:15). In other words, just like a weed, it lodges in your core, begins to choke the good in your life, and leads to unwanted outcomes. Bitterness causes unsuspecting, well-intentioned people trouble in all the areas that are key to overall health and wellness:

- *Spiritually.* When bitterness gets a foothold, you lose the ability to live in a place of praise, grace, and forgiveness. You begin to pull away from God, which gives bitterness the space to dig in even deeper. The more bitter you become, the harder it is to get those weeds out of your heart.

- *Mentally.* When you are harboring bitterness toward someone, unhealthy thoughts fill your mind. Bitterness begins directing your mind and, before long, your actions. The person you are having a conflict with may move across the country or even die, but the negativity you feel won't go with them unless you make an intentional choice to uproot it and let it go. Otherwise, it will continue to grow in your heart and play with your mind, destroying your ability to live the life God has for you.

- *Emotionally.* Lingering bitterness can cause significant problems for your emotional health. When you don't truly forgive someone who has hurt you, that unforgiveness not only taints your relationship with that person but also hinders your ability to authentically give yourself to the other people in your life. Afraid of getting hurt again, you become more guarded. You start constructing walls around your heart. Inevitably, you reach a place where trust, grace, and love take a backseat to self-preservation. When you are troubled emotionally, you can't engage with others as God would have you engage with them, you can't think clearly or be as passionate about your calling, and you are more likely to make poor choices in regard to your health. Again, every area is intertwined.

- *Physically.* Bitterness acts like poison in your body. While you may think it is just a heart and mind issue, it's not; its effects run much deeper. The negative emotions bitterness produces are a contributing factor to an array of diseases. According to one researcher at Concordia University, "When harbored for a long time, bitterness may forecast patterns of biological dysregulation, a physiological impairment that can affect metabolism, immune response or organ function and physical disease."[1]

Bitterness and unforgiveness cause specific biological reactions within the body that include adrenaline and cortisol secretions, immune suppression, and increased blood pressure. Elevated cortisol levels tend to cause fat deposition in the abdominal area that is referred to as *toxic fat*. As the name suggests, this fat is linked to the development of cardiovascular diseases, including heart attacks and strokes. Since toxic emotions lead to toxic fat, letting go of bitterness and learning to forgive are not only helpful for weight loss but could also save your life.

Toxic emotions lead to toxic fat.

Strategies for Keeping Bitterness Away

Your body was not created to carry bitterness. Allowing the negative emotion to linger is like drinking a poisonous concoction. You may not feel the effects at first, but over time, they will destroy you. Therefore, learning to avoid and overcome bitterness is key to living a happy, healthy life. Here are some strategies for keeping bitterness away.

Expect Painful Relationships

Your relationships with other people will be the source of both your greatest pleasure and your greatest pain. No one is perfect—and it shows when we get close to one another. Take a look at what the prophet Jeremiah wrote: "The human heart is the most deceitful of all things, and desperately wicked. Who really knows how bad it is?" (Jer. 17:9).

We are all flawed. We are going to let one another down. We will disappoint one another. We will make one another angry.

The grace of God is the only thing that keeps hurtful failings and disappointments from happening any more than they do.

Since we are all imperfect human beings, we have to learn to expect pain in relationships. If we think our connections with other people are going to be rosy all the time, we are setting ourselves up for major disillusionment. We end up surprised when something hurtful happens, so we are more likely to respond with anger—which can trigger unforgiveness and plant the seeds for bitterness.

On the other hand, when we acknowledge that every relationship is going to have its share of problems, we are prepared when they come along and can deal with them more effectively. We can address the issue rather than turn against the other person. Remember, sidestepping surprise is one of the keys to maintaining emotional well-being (see chapter 13).

The people closest to us are those who can hurt us most deeply and the ones it is most important for us to forgive. This has always been the case. Even King David dealt with the relational pain that comes with a close relationship.

> It is not an enemy who taunts me—
> 　　I could bear that.
> It is not my foes who so arrogantly insult me—
> 　　I could have hidden from them.
> Instead, it is you—my equal,
> 　　my companion and close friend.
> What good fellowship we once enjoyed
> 　　as we walked together to the house of God.
> 　　(Ps. 55:12 14)

David was dealing with trouble caused by a close friend. Some scholars even believe he was referring to his son. If King David, a man after God's own heart (Acts 13:22), had to deal with pain in his closest relationships, why would we think we could avoid it?

Pain is part of every relationship just as thorns are part of every rose. When you accept that reality, you will be better prepared to handle the pain well when it shows up.

Choose to Rely on God and Stay the Course

During one of the most emotionally difficult periods of my life, I (Nelson) was facing some circumstances that had me completely on the defensive. I felt as if I was being attacked from all sides and wanted nothing more than to give up and run. During that time, God kept bringing this passage to my mind:

> In my distress I prayed to the LORD,
> and the LORD answered me and set me free.
> The LORD is for me, so I will have no fear.
> What can mere people do to me?
> Yes, the LORD is for me; he will help me.
> I will look in triumph at those who hate me.
> It is better to take refuge in the LORD
> than to trust in people. (Ps. 118:5–8)

Reminding myself of this passage helped me recenter my mind on truth. Think about the words "What can mere people do to me? The LORD is for me." When you are able to keep that perspective and lean into your reliance on God, hurtful situations with those around you lose much of their sting. God gives you the strength to stand and face whatever you are going through, deal with it as it should be dealt with, and move on with a clear, healthy mind and heart.

As part of this, remember that nothing gets resolved without humility. As you rely on God in painful situations, it is important to have a high degree of humility. Whenever there is strife, our natural tendency is to blow up with pride and defend ourselves, try to prove that we are right, and insinuate that our perspective is the one most aligned with the way God thinks. What arrogance.

To keep bitterness from taking root in your heart, make humble a verb. Actively choose to let go of your need to be right. Be intentional about trying to see and understand things from the other person's point of view. Decide to love, in spite of the circumstances. For God to be able to work in the situation and stop bitterness from seeping into your heart, you must be willing to humble yourself, rely deeply on him, and stay the course in the relationship.

Forgive the People Who Hurt You

Forgiveness. It is not always easy, is it? But as difficult as forgiving those who hurt you can be, doing so is crucial to your well-being. It is necessary if you ever hope to experience the fullness of life God has planned for you. After all, forgiveness isn't a suggestion; it's a command: "Make allowance for each other's faults, and forgive anyone who offends you. Remember, the Lord forgave you, so *you must forgive others*" (Col. 3:13, emphasis added). Scripture says we *must* forgive others. There are no caveats or qualifiers—just the simple instruction to do it.

> *The consequence of not forgiving others and allowing a root of bitterness to grow inside you is much more costly to you than it is to the one against whom you are harboring negative emotions.*

According to a study at Virginia Commonwealth University, chronic unforgiveness causes physical harm to the body. Every time you think of the person who wronged you, your body responds with powerful chemical reactions. Forgiving, on the other hand, actually strengthens your immune system. The consequence of not forgiving others and allowing a root of bitterness to grow inside you is much more costly to you than it is to the one against whom you are harboring negative emotions.

Still, forgiveness is difficult, especially when the wounds are deep. But one of the reasons it is so hard is that we misunderstand the true nature of forgiveness. We tend to think it is something it's not. Here is what forgiveness is not:

- saying that someone's actions were justified
- denying how much you were hurt
- something that hinges on you receiving an apology first

Would internalizing these realities make it easier for you to forgive someone who hurt you? You are not saying the person's actions were okay. You are not denying your own pain. And you are not at the mercy of whether or not they decide to apologize. Instead, you are proactively choosing to let go of unforgiveness and bitterness for your own benefit. If you don't, that thing you are upset about will continue to hold power over you, influence your life, and harm your health.

The Process of Biblical Forgiveness

Once you understand what forgiveness is not, forgiving becomes easier. But how exactly do you go about it? You can begin by working through the three-step process of biblical forgiveness:

1. Remember How Much You Have Been Forgiven
2. Release the Person Who Hurt You
3. Reestablish the Relationship, as Much as Possible

Let's take a closer look at each of the three steps in this process.

Remember How Much You Have Been Forgiven

If you are struggling to forgive someone who hurt you, pause and remember just how much God has forgiven you. Think about the magnitude of God's grace in your own life. Think about

144

Jesus and the cross. Think about the gift of forgiveness he offers to every person walking the earth, no matter what they have done, no matter how undeserving.

Grasping the extent of God's grace in your own life is the only thing that will give you the ability to show astonishing grace to others. Bitterness is a natural response when you have been wounded; forgiveness is supernatural. God alone gives you the power to forgive the seemingly unforgivable as you recognize the work he has done in your life and in the lives of those you love.

> *Grasping the extent of God's grace in your own life is the only thing that will give you the ability to show astonishing grace to others.*

Release the Person Who Hurt You

Releasing someone who hurt you means letting that person out of the prison you have constructed for them in your mind. It means making a decision to stop dwelling on how they did you wrong and intentionally letting go of any bitterness that has worked its way into your heart. To get there, hand the situation and all the emotions associated with it over to God. Trust him to deal with it in the proper way. After all, he is much better equipped to handle these things. Once you choose to release your offender, you will experience a huge sense of peace and comfort.

This step is not easy. Holding on to the hurt can make you feel as if you are paying the person who offended you back for what they did. But you aren't. Harboring anger and bitterness doesn't do anything except allow the situation to continue holding you hostage, wreaking havoc on you physically, emotionally, and spiritually. While you may not *feel* like releasing the person who caused you pain, understand that this step is a proactive choice rather than the result of a feeling—and it is a choice necessary for your own healing and future well-being.

Reestablish the Relationship, as Much as Possible

Forgiveness and reconciliation are not the same thing. Forgiveness is a requirement for moving past pain in a healthy way, but reconciliation has to be considered on a case-by-case basis. As Paul wrote, "Do all that you can to live in peace with everyone" (Rom. 12:18).

You can do your part by remembering how much you have been forgiven, releasing the other person, and doing what you can to prayerfully reestablish the relationship. But keep in mind that some relationships can't or shouldn't be reestablished. For example, don't reconnect in a relationship that may cause you additional personal harm or expose you to any kind of emotional or physical danger. Be wise. Forgiveness doesn't require putting yourself back in a questionable situation. (For more on forgiveness, go to NewYouBook.com.)

If you are going to avoid bitterness and all its negative effects, you are going to have to become a good forgiver. You will have to repeat the process many times as you move through life. So one of the greatest things you can do for your health and well-being is to make being quick to forgive a habit—a reflex, even. Practice generous forgiveness every chance you get. Consider this passage: "Then Peter came to him and asked, 'Lord, how often should I forgive someone who sins against me? Seven times?' 'No, not seven times,' Jesus replied, 'but seventy times seven!'" (Matt. 18:21–22).

Keeping the Weeds Away

Do you have a lot of weeding to do in the garden of your life? Do you have some roots of bitterness that need to be pulled? Remember, just like gardening, letting go of unforgiveness and bitterness is hard, backbreaking work, but it is work that must be done, work that is essential to your health on every level, work that will help cultivate a beautiful new you, ready to showcase God's excellence to the world.

Small Steps to the New You

1. Ask God to help you identify specific areas of bitterness in your heart.

2. Make a list of the people you need to forgive and pray for the strength to do so.

3. Forgive one person who hurt you using the process for biblical forgiveness. Then another person. Then another.

4. Get out in the yard and do some weeding (if the season permits). It will solidify the image of uprooting bitterness—and give you some exercise to boot!

16

the sleep connection

Why Sleep Is Vitally Important
and How to Get More of It

Sleep is a key element of our well-being and interacts profoundly with each of the other parts.

Arianna Huffington

God gives rest to his loved ones.

Psalm 127:2

Have you ever thought of sleep as being as important to your health as the food you eat and the amount of exercise you get? That is not how we usually think of sleep, is it? We think of it as something we can get by with less of, something negotiable. We even wear a lack of sleep like a badge of honor, feeling as if skimping makes us look busier and more productive than the next person. But all this wrong thinking about sleep is only getting us sick, making us fatter, clouding our minds, and frying our emotions.

If you want to become the new you that you are envisioning—if you want to walk in the fullness of all God has for you—it is time to take another look at sleep. Sleep is not a luxury. Making sure you get seven to eight hours each night is not an indulgence. Quite the opposite. Sleep is a nonnegotiable component of overall wellness. Without healthy sleep, your health will suffer in every way.

The Importance of Sleep

Your body was crafted for sleep. When God knit you together, he fashioned your systems in such a way that they need deep rest in order to function properly. Without sleep, breakdown begins.

Don't take it from us; with every passing year, more and more scientific evidence emerges to underscore the importance of quality sleep. Study after study shows that sleep is critical to good health, while sleep deprivation is linked to increased risks of the following:

- diabetes
- cancer
- heart attack
- obesity
- stroke
- Alzheimer's disease[1]

Not to mention, a lack of sleep destroys your ability to function at your best on a daily basis.

Here are just a few of the benefits of good sleep.

Improved Clarity

When you get a good night's rest, you have more energy the following day. You think more clearly and make better decisions. One extensive study concluded that people who get eight hours

149

of sleep each night are significantly more focused and better able to perform tasks than those who get six hours of sleep.[2] Six hours of sleep was shown to lead to cognitive decline, which resulted in poor decision making, poor reactions to stimuli, and compromised productivity. Scarily, the average American subsists on around six hours of sleep each night.[3]

For years, I (Nelson) tried to convince myself that I could do fine on five to six hours of sleep, but as I became a student of this subject and committed to getting more rest, I realized I had been living an illusion. I had been compromising my work while telling myself I was getting more done. That doesn't make a lot of sense, does it? My life was suffering because I wouldn't give my body the sleep it required. Is yours?

Lower Stress

Sleep is God's prescription for minimizing stress and keeping you emotionally healthy. When you are in a stressed state, the cortisol (your body's stress hormone) levels in your system surge. Over time, continually high levels of cortisol lead to immunity suppression, weight gain, stomach problems, heart problems, and more. Sleep is one of the main ways your body neutralizes that stress hormone. When you go to sleep, your stress level begins to fall and your system has the opportunity to normalize. Getting a good night's rest is like hitting a reset button on your body. (For more on lowering stress, see chapter 17.)

> *Sleep is God's prescription for minimizing stress and keeping you emotionally healthy.*

Better Physical and Mental Health

Getting enough sleep is undeniably connected to physical health. For starters, a lack of sleep is directly tied to increased weight gain. In a study by the Mayo Clinic, sleep-restricted people gained more weight than their well-rested counterparts over the course of a week, consuming an average of 559 extra calories a day. People who get six hours of sleep per night are 23 percent more likely to be overweight. For people who get less than four hours of sleep per night, that percentage climbs to a staggering 73 percent.[4]

You might think it would take years of poor sleep habits for physical problems to start showing up. Not so. One study simulated the effects of the poor sleep patterns of shift workers on ten healthy young adults. After just four days of insufficient sleep, a third of them had glucose levels that qualified as prediabetic.[5]

Sleep is as important to mental health as it is to physical health. Good sleep allows the brain to shed toxins, including proteins that are associated with Alzheimer's disease. Plus, sleep deprivation has been found to have a strong connection to practically every mental health disorder we know of, especially depression and anxiety.[6]

Sleep is not something to be taken lightly. Your health literally depends on it. If you want to be well, you have to understand the life-giving benefits of sleep and learn to prioritize it in your life—because not doing so is so easy. As Arianna Huffington wrote in *The Sleep Revolution: Transforming Your Life One Night at a Time*, "The path of least resistance is the path of insufficient sleep. And unless we take specific and deliberate steps to make it a priority in our lives, we won't get the sleep we need."[7]

Making sleep a priority begins with adopting a new view of sleep.

A New View of Sleep

A few years ago, as I (Nelson) was studying Genesis in preparation for a teaching series, God brought something significant to my attention—a truth that became a paradigm-shifting revelation concerning my view of sleep. At first glance, the truth seems simple enough: when God created the world, he created the night before the day (Gen. 1:2–4). The darkness preceded the light. While this fact may seem insignificant on the surface, it is transformative when you follow it through.

In our culture, we consider nightfall the end of the day. We work hard through all our waking hours, and when the hour is finally late enough to justify our actions, we turn off all our screens and fall into bed exhausted. The next day begins when the alarm clock goes off. However, the Hebrew concept of night and day illustrated in Genesis is much different and arguably much more productive. In it, each sunset begins the preparation period for the next day. Sleep is not the reward for a day well spent; it is preparation for what God is calling you to tomorrow. In other words, tonight is not the end of today; it is the beginning of tomorrow.

This subtle change in perspective shifted my understanding of sleep. I began to realize that if God is going to accomplish what he wants to accomplish through me, I need to prepare myself by getting enough rest at night to be truly ready for what the next day will bring. My ability to fulfill my purpose is directly linked to how rested I am when I wake up each morning. The same is true for you.

> *Sleep is not the reward for a day well spent; it is preparation for what God is calling you to tomorrow.*

Nighttime sleep is the prep time you and I have been given for each new day. It is a gift. Taking sleep seriously is our way of saying, "God, I want to be ready for what you have for me. I don't want to miss or compromise your will because of my refusal to get the sleep I need to be at my best." Since I have learned to give sleep the place in my life it deserves, not only am I more pleasant to be around but I am also more effective in my calling than I ever was during those years when I tried to function on fumes.

How to Get More Sleep

Still, sometimes it is just hard to put down what we are doing and turn out the light. We are all guilty of what sleep scientists call bedtime procrastination. That is, we don't go to bed when we know we should because there is always one more thing to do—one more email to send, one more chapter to read, one more episode to watch. You know how it goes.

As with other areas of our health, we have to be intentional about getting our sleep to the level that will serve us best. Here are a few tips for breaking the procrastination cycle and getting more shut-eye.

Go to Bed Fifteen Minutes Earlier

You probably have a certain time you need to be up in the morning. Sleeping in isn't an option. So to start getting more sleep, you have to add it to the front end of the night. In other words, you have to go to bed earlier.

Try easing into an earlier bedtime. If you suddenly start going to bed an hour before you are used to, you may find yourself staring at the ceiling until your body adjusts. Instead, go to bed fifteen minutes earlier every night for a month. The next month, go to bed fifteen minutes earlier than that. Keep backing up your bedtime by fifteen minutes each month until you are getting seven to eight hours of sleep every night.

Create a Bedtime Routine

Parents know that kids go to sleep much easier when a predictable bedtime routine is in place. Maybe it involves a bath, changing into comfy pajamas, reading a book, or playing with a favorite toy. No matter the specifics, routine helps signal kids' bodies that sleep is coming. As adults, we usually lose this practice, but we shouldn't.

A wind-down routine will help you transition out of your hectic day and into sleep. Don't get too elaborate; just start doing something consistently that relaxes you and puts you in a sleepier state. Have a cup of herbal tea or read a few pages of a novel. Spend some time in quiet prayer. Do whatever helps you cross the divide from busy to bed.

Do a "Big Sleep" Two or Three Times Each Year

Sometimes the best thing you can do to accomplish more is to get some much-needed rest. That is the idea behind the big sleep—a concept we came across several years ago and have made great use of ever since.

Let's say it is Thursday afternoon. You are trying to pull things together for an upcoming weekend commitment, but because of side issues demanding your attention, unusual family situations, and a slew of other to-dos on your radar, you are having a hard time working through all that needs to be done. Your stress level is high; your anxiety is through the roof; you are overwhelmed and so far behind with everything that you aren't sure which way to turn next. At that moment, what should you do?

Here is what you shouldn't do. You shouldn't keep plowing through. You shouldn't stay up half the night to get everything done. Pushing harder isn't the answer. You will just start hitting your head against the ceiling of diminishing returns. Though it may seem counterintuitive at first, your best plan is to hit the reset button by doing a big sleep. Leave everything behind and go to bed for twelve full hours.

Sounds crazy, right? Trust us on this: the most effective way to clear your head and break the cycle of stress is to do a big sleep at the exact time you think there is no way you can afford to. Let your family in on your plan and then steal away for an extended night's rest. If you don't think you can physically sleep for twelve hours, use the first part of that time to unwind—alone and completely unplugged from technology. Take a walk or read a book, then get in bed nice and early. When you get up the next morning, you are going to be refocused, reenergized, and ready to tackle everything that seemed ready to tackle you the day before.

Now, you can't do a big sleep every night. But if you adopt the practice two to three times per year, when things seem particularly hectic and stressful, you will soon learn that a big sleep doesn't cost you any time or productivity. In fact, it doubles your time and productivity by giving you the ability to face your circumstances refreshed and clearheaded. After one or two successful big sleeps, you will understand why some of the most productive people in the world have made this a habit.

How Are You Sleeping?

Even when we understand the importance of prioritizing sleep, gauging whether we are getting enough can still be difficult. In the sleep study mentioned above—the one showing cognitive decline among those who got only six hours of sleep—most of the sleep-deprived participants insisted they were getting enough sleep and weren't being negatively affected by sleeping less than eight hours. But the research proved them wrong. They were significantly impaired. We are so conditioned to get by on too little sleep that we are not always the best judges of whether our needs are being met. To begin determining if you are getting enough sleep, ask yourself these questions:

- *How much sleep do I need?* While there are rare exceptions on both sides of the equation, most of us need approximately eight hours of sleep every night to function at our best. If you aren't sure whether you need the full eight hours, consider the following questions.

- *Am I waking up without an alarm?* If the answer is no, you probably aren't getting enough sleep. When you hit your sweet spot—you may still want to set an alarm to make sure you don't oversleep—you should wake up feeling rested sometime in the thirty minutes before it sounds. If you aren't, that is a sign you need to go to bed earlier.

- *Am I able to go to sleep within thirty minutes of lying down?* Over a few months, this question, combined with the one above, will help you figure out exactly how much sleep you need. If you know you aren't getting enough sleep but you are having problems falling asleep when you go to bed, try establishing a wind-down routine, as mentioned above. If you aren't able to go to sleep because your mind is consumed with worry, try giving your concerns over to God. Trust him enough to close your eyes and rest, knowing that you will be better able to face the next day if you do. God is going to be awake all night anyway. You can hand everything off to him to carry through the night. As King David wrote, "The one who watches over you will not slumber" (Ps. 121:3). Another thing that is helpful is to make a to-do list for the next day before you go to bed. That way you won't lie awake worrying about forgetting something you need to do.

- *Am I waking up rested and pain free?* When you wake up rested and pain free, you know you are getting quality sleep—and quality is just as important as quantity. If your answer to this question is no, you will have to do a little investigating to figure out why. Nine times out of ten, though, the mattress you are sleeping on is the biggest problem. An old or poor-quality mattress can cause disrupted sleep and back pain. The effects aren't worth the money you save by buying a cheap mattress or holding on to the same one for more than a decade. As your body ages and changes, so do your mattress needs. Take some time to explore what works

156

best for you. Personally, I (Nelson) saved up a few years ago and invested in one of the top-of-the-line memory foam mattresses; it revolutionized my sleep. Not only does it support my body with pressure at the right points so that I wake up rested and without pain but it also keeps my wife and me from waking each other up when we move around in the middle of the night. While an issue such as mattress quality may sound trivial at first, it is not. The more you do to make sure you are getting the rest you need, the better your health, your life, and your ability to fulfill God's plans will be.

- *Am I dozing off during the day?* If you are dozing off during the day, you probably aren't getting the quantity or quality of sleep you need at night. If you are struggling to stay awake only occasionally, then you should be able to address the problem by improving your sleep in the ways discussed here. But if you notice an ongoing problem—or if you are falling asleep in dangerous situations, such as while you are driving—talk to your doctor. Your drowsiness could be a sign of sleep apnea or some other condition that is keeping you from resting well at night.

Use these questions to help you figure out the current quality of your sleep and then do whatever it takes to begin getting the rest you need. Healthy people understand that sleep is a nonnegotiable component of overall well-being. Don't let the sleep-deprived culture we live in convince you otherwise.

Small Steps to the New You

1. Go to bed fifteen minutes earlier every night this month.
2. Invest in a better mattress or begin saving up to buy one in the future.
3. Try sleeping with a pillow between your knees to alleviate back pain.

small steps to better mental health

17

sidestepping stress

Practical Steps to Lower Your Anxiety

If you ask me what is the single most important key to longevity, I would have to say it is avoiding worry, stress and tension. And if you didn't ask me, I'd still have to say it.

George Burns

In this world you will have trouble. But take heart! I have overcome the world.

John 16:33 NIV

An old legend you may have heard tells about a man who worked for a major grocery store chain. During an overnight shift, he was working in the store's warehouse area by himself. He went into one of the freezer compartments to grab something he needed, and the freezer door accidentally closed behind him. He tried to get out, but he couldn't get the door to open. He was trapped.

Panicking, he yelled for his coworker, who was stocking shelves near the front of the store, but she couldn't hear him. He kicked and banged on the freezer door until his feet ached and his hands started to crack, but it wouldn't budge. Finally, he sat down on the floor of the freezer and took out a notepad he had in his pocket. He started recording what was happening to him. He wrote that he was beginning to feel cold and weak. He could feel his body freezing, he said. He scribbled that he didn't know if he would get out of the freezer alive.

The following morning, two store employees opened the freezer compartment and found the man lying on the floor, dead. The amazing part of the story? The freezer wasn't even that cold. It had started kicking on and off sporadically a few days earlier, so the compartment wasn't actually at freezing temperatures. But the trapped man believed it was. He believed he was freezing to death, and the stress his body underwent as a result turned that belief into reality. The cold didn't kill him; his own stress did.

The Stress-Health Connection

Walking in the fullness of the new you goes beyond eating well, exercising, and getting enough rest. To achieve and maintain true health, you also have to learn to handle the stress in your life. Otherwise, it will derail your other efforts, keeping you over-weight, sick, emotionally bound, and quite possibly taking you to an early grave.

When you begin to get stressed, your body reacts physically by going into what is known as fight-or-flight mode. This stress response causes your heart to race, your breathing to quicken, your muscles to contract, and your blood pressure to rise. Your body is literally preparing itself to act in the face of danger, even if that danger isn't physical. When you are in this state often, it wears your body down. Constant stress leads to weight gain, low energy, headaches, digestive issues, frequent colds and infections, premature aging, and a host of other problems.[1] Over the long term, it can cause heart disease, heart attacks, and an increased cancer risk.

While the physical effects of stress are nothing to be taken lightly, high levels of stress also affect your mental well-being. Stress causes you to lose clarity and make poor decisions. In fact, we would venture that the worst decisions you have made in your life were made when you were under a great deal of stress. Stress causes you to have a sour mood and a quick temper, which lead to countless relational issues. There is no margin in your life when you are stressed, so you tend to overreact to everything and hurt the people around you. (For a refresher on maintaining emotional strength, turn back to chapter 13.)

Not to mention, stress hinders your spiritual life. Have you noticed that when you are overwhelmed and feel you have too much to do, your prayer life is one of the first things to go? Your time in God's Word usually follows. This creates a vicious cycle. As your stress causes you to crowd God out of your schedule, you begin to lose the sense of his peace and presence—which you need more than ever when you are stressed. This loss causes even more stress, which makes you pull even farther away. Again, everything works together. No area of your life stands alone. (For a refresher on living a fully engaged spiritual life, turn back to chapter 9.)

Think of stress as something that maximizes whatever is going on in the rest of your life. When you are under high stress, the negative in your life is maximized—health problems, emotional discontent, spiritual distance, relational tension, and the list goes on. On the other hand, when you are managing your stress levels well and keeping them low, the good in your life is maximized. You are able to achieve better physical health, you are more emotionally stable, you have more mental clarity, and you are more invested in your relationships with God and other people.

Still, stress is an unavoidable part of life. You are never going to get away from it, so you have to learn to manage it. As Jesus said, "In this world you will have trouble. But take heart! I have overcome the world" (John 16:33 NIV). With this in mind, consider these two truths about stress:

- *There is no such thing as a stress-free life.* From the average person on the street to the president of the United States, everyone deals with some level of stress. As long as you are on this side of heaven, you are never going to be able to eliminate stress as a constant companion—but you can learn to manage and minimize it.

- *You are never going to get everything done.* One of the greatest sources of stress is the never-ending to-do list. There is always going to be another meeting to go to, another list to shop for, another budget to prepare, another doctor's appointment to squeeze in, another deadline to hit, another load of laundry to wash, another bill to pay— you get the idea. If you are like most people, you could tick things off your to-do list twenty-four hours a day for a week straight and still not get to the end of it. As soon as you mark one thing off, something else appears in its place, right? Knowing that you are never going to get everything done helps relieve some of the pressure you inevitably put on yourself.

When you acknowledge these two truths, they bring a modicum of peace. They confirm that you are not alone. You are not the only one dealing with high levels of stress. You are not the only one facing challenge after challenge in your life. You are not the only one with a to-do list that seems impossible to manage. These things are simply part of living a busy life.

Knowing stress is a common condition of humankind helps bring it into perspective. The difference between those who allow stress to eat them alive and those who stay cool under pressure isn't the actual level of stress they are under but how well they have learned to deal with its presence.

> *The difference between those who allow stress to eat them alive and those who stay cool under pressure isn't the actual level of stress they are under but how well they have learned to deal with its presence.*

Strategies for Successful Stress Management

Since stress is something we have to welcome into our lives and commit to managing well, we would be smart to streamline the stress management process as much as possible. Here are some simple tips for keeping your stress in check and making sure you don't end up freezing to death in a lukewarm freezer.

Understand the Difference between Good Stress and Bad Stress

Yes, there is such a thing as good stress. Small amounts of good stress keep you focused and motivated. You grow through certain levels of stress. The stress gravity exerts on you makes your bones denser and your muscles stronger. When you exercise, your endurance rises as a result of the stress you impose on yourself. When you decide to do something like read a book every month for your personal or professional growth, you are adding stress to your life, but it is productive stress—stress that will result in reward for you and those around you. Maximizing the good stress in your life is a wise thing to do. In fact, it is necessary for positive change.

Stress becomes bad when it passes the point of growing you and distresses you instead. Perhaps the phone rings, and suddenly there is a problem you didn't see coming. Perhaps you realize you are way over budget, and there is not much time to get caught up. The key to handling bad stress is to continually grow your threshold for dealing with it. Some people freak out at the first sign of a negative issue, while others can take the same issue in stride. The difference is their tolerance threshold for stress. Growing that threshold will enable you to deal with bad stress without, well, stressing out. The next few tips will help you do just that.

Get Clear on the Source of Your Stress

A lack of clarity raises your stress level. When a difficult situation tries to send you over the edge, ask yourself exactly what about that situation is so bothersome. Then address the source of the stress rather than wallowing in the stress itself. Worrying is often just a result of being unclear about your next step. When you can identify the source of your problem, you will usually know what to do about it. You can't always control the situation you find yourself in, but you can control your perception of and response to the situation—and that can make all the difference in the world in your stress level.

> You can't always control the situation you find yourself in, but you can control your perception of and response to the situation.

Manage Your Time Well

There is a major correlation between high stress and a perceived lack of time. If you manage your time poorly, you will always struggle under the pressure of having more to do than there are hours in the day. On the other hand, by learning to manage your time well, you will be able to exponentially increase your ability to tolerate stress. Here are a couple of key tips for managing your time in a way that helps keep stress down:

- *Don't start the day until you finish the day.* Stress is often an indicator that something in your life is out of control. To regain some of that control, make a practice of finishing the day (in terms of thoughts and planning) before you start it. In other words, sketch out how your day is going to look. Review your to-do list and add what needs to be added. You can do this before bed the night before, as mentioned in the last chapter, if doing so will help you clear your mind. Or you can do it first thing in the morning before you kick off your day. Find what works best for you. Then review your list, prioritize your most important tasks, and tackle those tasks first. Which leads to . . .

- *Eat the frog.* As you look at your to-do list for the day, decide to eat the frog on the list first thing. In other words, do the hardest thing on your list first so that it won't be hanging over your head and weighing on you for the rest of the day. Otherwise, you will procrastinate on that thing. You will let that frog sit close by and blow you kisses all day long while you try to check off other items you enjoy more than frog eating. Getting the frog out of the way first thing in the morning will lower your stress and increase your overall productivity for the day. So whether the task is tackling a project you have been putting off, making a difficult phone call, or any number of things that may be filling you with dread, just do it . . . eat the frog. Once it is down, you will be so glad you did.

- *Live off peak.* Eliminating wait time in your life will help you eliminate stress. One of the best ways to do that is to commit to an off-peak lifestyle. If you are someone who has a flexible schedule, take advantage of that flexibility to cut down on the amount of time you spend doing the things everyone

167

does—like grocery shopping, going to the post office, eating out—and then add those saved minutes and hours back into other areas of your day. For example, if you are planning a lunch meeting at a restaurant, schedule it for before or after the usual lunchtime rush hour. This simple step could save you thirty minutes. If you have to go to the bank, don't go close to five o'clock when the rest of the world will be there. Go at a random time in the afternoon and prevent waiting from eating away at your day. You will accomplish the task and save yourself precious time in the process. Simple steps such as these have the potential to lower your stress level significantly.

Practice Positive Self-Talk

Think of the stress in your life as a flame. When it flares up, you can do one of two things. You can either throw gasoline on it to make it rage even harder or drench it with water. The internal monologue running in your head will act as either gas or water. Again, you can't always control the stressful situations in your life, but you can control your response to them. Part of that is controlling what you say to yourself about those situations. The story running in your head will either make the stress worse than it needs to be or help shrink it down to a manageable level.

The story running in your head will either make the stress worse than it needs to be or help shrink it down to a manageable level.

You have more power to control your stress than you think. Don't reinforce the chaos in your life by saying things to yourself such as the following:

- I'm so stressed out.
- I'm just overwhelmed.

- I can't believe this is happening.
- I'm so far behind; I'm never going to get this done.

This kind of negative self-talk keeps the flame raging. Take those thoughts captive and choose instead to see a more positive side of your situation.

Praise God for the work he has given you to do. Praise him that he blesses you with the strength and clarity of mind to handle everything he brings your way. Talk to yourself about how good it is going to feel to eat your next frog. Focus on all that you are getting done. In short, when you talk to yourself, choose your words wisely. (Much more on this in the next chapter.)

Take Mini Breaks throughout the Day

One of the best ways to get ahead of stress is to step back from the situations that are stressing you. When you feel your tension level getting high, take a little break. Doing so will slow the momentum of a stressful situation and keep it from spiraling out of control.

Say someone shoots you a not-so-nice email that sends your stress level soaring. Instead of immediately sending an emotionally driven email back or picking up the phone and calling that person while you are upset, step back. Literally move away from your computer or put down your phone and take some deep breaths. Go for a short walk. Use those few minutes to pray about the situation. This kind of mini break will give you more perspective and allow you to respond from a calmer place. Otherwise, you will just fuel the fire and make things worse.

On a related note, use your transition times throughout the day as mini breaks—as small opportunities to decompress. Don't carry stress from one task to the next. Take a mini break in between so you are more refreshed for the next thing coming down the track. For example, start thinking of your drive to pick up the kids or your drive home in the evening as a mini break. It is your chance to step out of the stress and busyness of the day and clear your head before reconnecting with your family. Listen to some praise music as you drive or do something else that helps you find your way to a more peaceful place. Learn to use these mini breaks to leave each stressor where it belongs rather than carrying cumulative tension through your entire day.

Praise God during Times of Stress

Praising God when things are going well is easy, but how quick are you to praise him when you feel overwhelmed? When your stress level is high, practice praising God for giving you the opportunity to grow. Let the strain you feel be a reminder to worship God for all he is doing in you and through you. As you do, God will use this practice to make you physically, spiritually, emotionally, and mentally healthier. You will be better able to sidestep the negative effects of stress while embracing all that God has in store for you in the future.

Small Steps to the New You

1. Remind yourself as often as necessary that stress is a natural, unavoidable part of life.

2. Make your to-do list either before you go to sleep at night or first thing in the morning.

3. Practice eating frogs and living off peak.

4. When you are in a season that feels particularly stressful, set a timer every hour to remind you to think about the good in your life and to praise God for his faithfulness.

18

the voice in your head

How Choosing the Right Thoughts
Can Change Your Life

Watch your thoughts; they become words.

Frank Outlaw

May the words of my mouth
    and the meditation of my heart
be pleasing to you,
    O LORD, my rock and my redeemer.

Psalm 19:14

Go to any metropolitan city in the world—and even some not so metropolitan—and you will inevitably see someone walking down the street talking to themselves. Your tendency, like ours, is probably to pity them for being disturbed as you watch their one-sided conversation out of the corner of your eye. The irony is that we all carry on conversations with ourselves all the time—just not usually out loud. Sometimes we may not even realize we are doing it. But whether we are aware of it or not, we talk to ourselves all day every day through the thoughts we allow to consume our minds.

Even if you have never keyed into them, your conscious and subconscious thoughts are your constant companions. They drive and form your every waking moment. How you choose to direct your thoughts will ultimately define your life. As James Allen wrote in the classic work on this topic, *As a Man Thinketh*:

> Man is made or unmade by himself; in the armory of thought he forges the weapons by which he destroys himself; he also fashions the tools with which he builds for himself heavenly mansions of joy and strength and peace. By the right choice and true application of thought, man ascends to the Divine Perfection; by the abuse and wrong application of thought, he descends below the level of the beast. Between these two extremes are all the grades of character, and man is their maker and master.[1]

You are made or unmade by your thoughts. Day after day, month after month, year after year, they create every condition of your life, so much so that situations and circumstances you perceive as happening *to* you are usually happening *because of* you, in one way or another. That is a tough pill to swallow, isn't it? No matter what the current state of your life is, your cumulative thoughts have largely landed you there. And every day they either keep you where you are, pull you backward, or propel you into a better future.

You are made or unmade by your thoughts.

The good news is that you get to choose whether what goes on in your head works for you or against you. You have the capacity to maximize the thoughts that are beneficial to your health, your success, your relationships, your faith, and every other area of your life and to disregard those that could keep you from attaining the full measure of what God has for you. This powerful reality has been co-opted and skewed in the past by nonbiblical thinkers, but, in its original form, it was God's idea. He not only gives us the power to control our thoughts and to use them to cooperate with his plan for us but also tells us to do just that, as we will see later in this chapter.

Cooperate with God in changing the voice in your head, and your whole life will reflect the change.

Your dominating thoughts create your reality. How? First, they fashion your beliefs. Valid or not, those beliefs shape your attitudes about yourself and the world around you. Your attitudes create your feelings, and your feelings drive the actions you take in every area of your life.[2] The way you see yourself and the world around you is an outgrowth of what goes on in your mind. Everything you choose to do or not do, say or not say, starts with the seed of thought. As a result, getting a handle on the voice no one hears but you is nonnegotiable when it comes to maximizing your mental health and stepping into the new you. Cooperate with God in changing the voice in your head, and your whole life will reflect the change.

Growing the Good

Think again about the idea of sowing and reaping. As we have discussed, your harvest in life will be the result of the type and quality of the seeds you plant in every area. Your mind is no exception. Each one of your thoughts is a seed that will, eventually, reap a harvest. What kind of harvest that will be is determined by the kind of seeds you sow. The very life you live is the bounty of your thoughts, its makeup completely determined by what you choose to plant in your mind. Along these lines, James Allen went on to write the following:

Man's mind may be likened to a garden, which may be intelligently cultivated or allowed to run wild; but whether cultivated or neglected, it must, and will, bring forth. If no useful seeds are put into it, then an abundance of useless weed-seeds will fall therein, and will continue to produce their kind. Just as a gardener cultivates his plot, keeping it free from weeds, and growing the flowers and fruits which he requires, so may a man tend the garden of his mind, weeding out all the wrong, useless, and impure thoughts, and cultivating toward perfection the flowers and fruits of right, useful, and pure thoughts. By pursuing this process, a man sooner or later discovers that he is the master-gardener of his soul, the director of his life. He also reveals, within himself, the laws of thought, and understands, with ever-increasing accuracy, how the thought-forces and mind elements operate in the shaping of his character, circumstances, and destiny.[3]

The thoughts you think act as instructions to your brain; as soon as they come through, your brain goes to work to turn them into reality. Or in keeping with the analogy, when you plant seeds of thought—no matter what kind of seeds they are—your brain gets busy producing a corresponding crop. Your subconscious mind can't differentiate between useful seeds and "weed-seeds" or between what is true and beneficial to you and what is not. It simply listens to the thoughts running around in your head, takes them at face value, and begins the process of growing them. That being the case, you need to step back and think about what you are saying to yourself and make sure you are using words that will reap a harvest of peace, joy, and fulfillment rather than the opposite.

There are three main areas of life where your thoughts produce an obvious, measurable return: your personal accomplishments, your relationships, and your health. Let's look at how each one of these areas is inextricably tied to what you say when you talk to yourself.

174

Your Thoughts and Your Personal Accomplishments

Every accomplishment in your life—whether it is how well you do in school, what level you hit in your professional life, or how you manage your household—is directly linked to how you feel about yourself, to whether you think you are capable and worthy of living life at the highest level. And what drives your evaluation of your abilities and worth? What you say about yourself when you talk to yourself or, as author Stephen Covey likes to put it, the mental script you operate from.[4]

Your mental script has been developing since the day you were born. It began with what your parents said to you. If your parents made comments that led you to believe you weren't smart enough, cute enough, or good enough, those hurtful words and the emotions that accompanied them started setting the foundation for how you see yourself. Along the way, friends, teachers, and personal experiences built on that foundation, shaping how you think about yourself and thereby shaping what you think you can do and be in this world. What you believe about yourself determines how you feel about yourself, how you feel about yourself dictates your daily actions, and your daily actions added up over time determine your level of accomplishment in the areas of life that are important to you.

When you wake up to this reality, you can begin to filter the contents of your mental script through the sieve of truth, keeping what is helpful and discarding what is not—a process that is crucial to creating a mental atmosphere that will allow you to operate at the full potential God has put in you. If you don't, you will end up living out your story based on the incomplete and often inaccurate script that has been handed to you by others. As Stephen Covey wrote:

> These scripts come from people, not principles. And they rise out of our deep vulnerabilities, our deep dependency on others and

our needs for acceptance and love, for belonging, for a sense of importance, for a feeling that we matter. Whether we are aware of it or not, whether we are in control of it or not, there is a first creation to every part of our lives. We are either the second creation of our own proactive design, or we are the second creation of other people's agenda, of circumstances or of past habits.[5]

Becoming "the second creation of [your] own proactive design" requires that you become aware of how you think about your value, your abilities, your dreams, and your goals; get rid of misinformation that isn't helping you live as the person you know you can be; and focus instead on your true identity as a new creation in Christ. Consider just a handful of Scripture passages that speak to who you really are:

For we are God's masterpiece. He has created us anew in Christ Jesus, so we can do the good things he planned for us long ago. (Eph. 2:10)

God created human beings in his own image. In the image of God he created them. (Gen. 1:27)

For you created my inmost being;
    you knit me together in my mother's womb.
I praise you because I am fearfully and wonderfully made.
    (Ps. 139:13–14 NIV)

See how very much our Father loves us, for he calls us his children, and that is what we are! (1 John 3:1)

Do you not know that you are the temple of God and that the Spirit of God dwells in you? (1 Cor. 3:16 NKJV)

"For I know the plans I have for you," says the LORD. "They are plans for good and not for disaster, to give you a future and a hope." (Jer. 29:11)

When you think negatively about yourself, you are putting down God. You are his child, created in his image. He knit you together with meticulous care, filled you with potential, and has given you everything you need to accomplish the purposes he has for you. Why, then, would you choose to spend precious time operating from a place of self-doubt and pessimism that will do nothing but undermine the level of your life?

You get to decide what mental script you allow to direct your thoughts and dictate your days—the script that has come to you from well-intentioned (perhaps) but often misguided people speaking out of their own poor scripts or a script based on the true identity God has given you as his child. Choose wisely. Your decision will determine the messages your subconscious mind receives and thereby control the direction and quality of your entire life.

Your Thoughts and Your Relationships

Your thought life manifests itself in the quality of your relationships with others. That is because how you think and feel about yourself dictates how you interact with people. For example, if you see yourself as shy or socially awkward, that belief will lead you to avoid social situations and lose out on the relationships you may find through them. If you avoid connecting with other people because you are afraid you won't be liked or that you will get hurt, you are crippling your life based on fear—fear that is counter to who you were created to be and perpetuated by the words you allow to run around in your head. Do you ever find yourself thinking things such as the following:

- I always say the wrong thing when I talk to them.
- I don't get along well with other people.
- Relationships are hard for me.
- I'm so uncomfortable in social settings.

177

Phrases like these put you on the path to relational frustration. They become self-fulfilling prophecies. You may very well say the wrong thing when you talk to people, but if you do it because you expect to, you are living by the mental script that mandates it. If you have told yourself that you are not good at relating to other people or maintaining long-term relationships, your subconscious is working to fulfill those thought patterns. If it hears you say, "Oh, I always feel so awkward in large groups of people," then guess what? You will dread the next social gathering you are invited to and then not enjoy it once you are there.

On the other hand, if you shift what you say when you talk to yourself and instead think things such as, *I love being with and talking with the people in my life, I'm thankful that I am able to connect with others and express myself clearly, I'm open to relationships*, or *I'm comfortable being myself and accepting others for who they are*, the way you engage with other people will change. Your subconscious will follow the new instructions and turn them into reality just as easily as it followed the old. With some time and repetition, the process really is that simple.

You can sabotage your relational life not only by thinking the wrong things about yourself but also by dwelling on the wrong thoughts when it comes to other people. For example, do you ever think things such as the following:

- My mother and I have so many issues; I don't think we'll ever work through them.
- My spouse and I just don't get along like we used to.
- My friends are so annoying. Why do I even spend time with them?

Thoughts like these may have truth to them. You and your mother may have complicated, deep-seated issues. But if you want to build your relationship with her, you can't let those issues dominate your thinking. Instead, make a decision to focus on the good in your relationship. Think about what you love about her. Talk to yourself about those things. An intentionally renewed focus will change not only the way you see her but also the way you talk to her. Over time, your relationship will be transformed for the better because you made a choice to direct your thoughts in a positive way rather than letting them carry you down the path to aggravating problems.

The same is true with your spouse, your children, your friends, and your coworkers. You will see what you are looking for. If you constantly think about the problems in your relationships or the shortcomings of the people around you, you will see only those problems and shortcomings as you interact with them. If you focus instead on the good in the people in your life, you will start to see that good manifest itself. This simple tweak will shift your entire perspective, strengthening and growing even your toughest relationships.

Your Thoughts and Your Health

How do you feel today? Are you tired? Are you sick? Maybe you are feeling healthy, happy, and on top of the world. Here is something that may surprise you: how you feel has almost everything to do with how you think you feel. If you wake up in the morning thinking about how tired you are and wishing you could just pull the covers over your head and stay put, you will start the day feeling sluggish. Your body will respond to the directive of your thoughts by dragging through the morning, sans energy. Your entire day may play out at a subpar level because of the mental atmosphere you created for yourself before you even got out of bed.

On the other hand, if you wake up choosing to be grateful for another morning, focusing on how healthy you are becoming and the promise the day holds, your body will again respond accordingly. You will move through your day with more energy and joy. You will feel better, look better, be able to stick to a healthy lifestyle better, and have more to offer those around you—and all because of what you chose to say to yourself when the alarm went off.

How you feel has almost everything to do with how you think you feel.

What goes on in your mind actually creates chemical realities within your body. Different thoughts and their accompanying emotions cause neurons to fire in your brain, setting off correlating physical reactions. This isn't new information. King David wrote about it thousands of years ago: "A cheerful heart is good medicine, but a broken spirit saps a person's strength" (Prov. 17:22).

Dr. Norman Vincent Peale took it a step further:

> The longer I live the more I am convinced that neither age nor circumstance needs to deprive us of energy and vitality. We are at last awakening to the close relationship between religion and health. We are beginning to comprehend a basic truth hitherto neglected, that our physical condition is determined very largely by our emotional condition, and our emotional life is profoundly regulated by our thought [mental] life. All through its pages, the Bible talks about vitality and force and life. The supreme over- all word of the Bible is life, and life means vitality—to be filled with energy.[6]

Science backs up both King David's and Peale's assertions. The stress that comes along with wrong thinking (and the resulting negative feelings and bad attitudes) raises blood pressure and re- leases cortisol into your system. We have already examined just how dangerous that can be over time. Choosing to let negative thoughts go in favor of more positive ones automatically improves your body's state of being, leading to more complete health and wellness. Filling your mind with the right thoughts is imperative to becoming the new you.

Thinking about Thinking

Since the quality of your life is so directly tied to the quality of your internal dialogue, you must do all you can to shape that dialogue for your own good. Understanding the power of your thoughts or knowing you need to change is not enough. You have to take specific action. Here are some practical steps you can take to help adopt better thinking.

Listen to Your Internal Dialogue

The first step to creating a healthier thought life doesn't require you to do anything but listen. You have to become aware of the script that is constantly running in your head.

One of the main things that separates us from the animals is our ability to think about our thought life, to note an individual thought passing through our minds, analyze it for its truth and worth, and then act accordingly. God gave us this unique ability when he made us in his image. But so often, we let our thoughts run on autopilot. They are just there, and we don't give them much consideration. Or worse, we forget that we are the masters of our own thoughts and let them have their way with us. As you begin tuning into your own mental environment, keep these basic truths about thoughts in mind:

- You can't always control the thoughts that pop into your head, but you can control what you do with them.

- Thoughts have only as much power as you give them. The more you dwell on a certain thought, the more powerful it will become.

- It is not a sin to have a wrong, negative, or tempting thought pass through your mind—if you let it pass right on through.

181

The sin comes when you choose to indulge that thought either by dwelling on it or acting on it.

Becoming aware of what is going on in your head is a good first step. Next, you have to take some action in response to what you hear.

Take Every Thought Captive

As you surrender yourself to God, he begins to fill you with more peace, love, and joy. But the positive effects of those gifts will be thwarted if you don't let them take root and influence your thoughts. It is up to you to resist habitual thought patterns and instead match your brain to the new thing God is doing in you.

How? By taking two steps Paul outlined in his letters to early Christian believers. The first step is to "take captive every thought to make it obedient to Christ" (2 Cor. 10:5 NIV). This starts with listening to the thoughts in your head, but it goes further. You have to evaluate your thoughts, trapping and disposing of the ones that don't line up with God's truth.

You can't always control the thoughts that pop into your head, but you can control what you do with them.

Second, Paul says to "fix your thoughts on what is true, and honorable, and right, and pure, and lovely, and admirable. Think about things that are excellent and worthy of praise" (Phil. 4:8). Paul says to "fix your thoughts." In other words, be proactive in choosing how you focus your thoughts. When you capture and get rid of thoughts that are not in line with what God is working in your heart and then follow that up by shifting your attention to things that are true, right, and excellent, you will begin to see yourself and the world around you differently. Your self-image will improve, your relationships will become stronger, your body will be healthier. And that is all before words even begin coming out of your mouth.

There is one more key ingredient to making this shift—something that has to happen in the space between these two steps, causing them to work together to become a lifestyle rather than just a short-term fix.

Replace Old Thinking with New

Psychologists tell us that we can't just get rid of a bad habit, including a negative thought pattern. We have to fill the vacated space with something new. Otherwise, our well-intentioned change won't last; we will revert right back to comfortable habits and well-worn patterns. So as you begin eliminating thoughts that don't benefit you, you have to immediately replace those thoughts with new ones that do. As you ship out the internal dialogue that keeps you depressed, shy, anxious, tired, and worried, you have to immediately fill the space in your mind that those thoughts occupied with a corresponding positive internal dialogue. It is not enough to think about true, positive, pure, and excellent things in general. Instead, connect them immediately to the vacated space of your captured thoughts. If you don't, those old thoughts will creep right back in.

One leading author on the topic explains this concept by describing the mind as a mental apartment furnished with the things you think about yourself and the world around you.

> [This furniture] is the old negative way of thinking that was handed down to us from our parents, our friends, our teachers. They gave us the furniture which we have kept and which we use in our mental apartment. Now let's say that I agree to come over and help you get rid of all the old furniture. We remove every piece, every dish, every rug, table, bed, sofa and chair. We take out every old negative self-belief and store it away safely out of sight.

183

After I leave, you stand in the middle of your mental apartment. You look around and think, "This is great! I've gotten rid of all my old negative thinking." . . . A little later that evening, after spending an hour or two with nothing but yourself and an empty apartment, what do you suppose you will do? You will go out to the garage where the old furniture is stored and get a chair! A little later, you will make another trip to the garage and bring in a table. . . . One by one you will begin to bring your old trusted and time-worn negative thoughts back into your mental apartment! Why? Because when I helped you remove the old furniture I didn't give you any new furniture to replace it with.

When you decide to stop thinking negatively, and do not have an immediate, new positive vocabulary to replace the old, you will always return to the comfortable, old, negative self-talk of the past.[7]

Think back to the relationship examples above. When negative, defeating thoughts about your parents, your spouse, your children, or anyone else pop up, it is not enough to simply say to yourself, *Oh, I shouldn't think such a thing*. Instead, you have to shift your focus toward something good, as we discussed. The most effective way to do that is to immediately replace the unproductive thought with a corresponding positive one. Out with the old, in with the new.

For example, if you catch yourself thinking something unconstructive, such as *I can't stand the way my children always second-guess me*, capture that thought, get rid of it, and then immediately fill the space with a better thought, such as *My children are learning to question and discern things for themselves. How can I nurture that?* Don't just stop at getting rid of the unhealthy thought; if you do, it will come back again and again. Instead, put something new in its place. Maybe you can see yourself in some of these examples:

Old thinking: I feel so fat and unhealthy.
Replacement thought: My body is an amazing machine. I am healthy and well.

Old thinking: I'm always tired.
Replacement thought: I feel great. I have so much energy today.

Old thinking: I'm sick of my job.
Replacement thought: I'm thankful for my job and the income it creates.

Old thinking: I'm not talented enough to do what I really want to do.
Replacement thought: I'm blessed with incredible skills and abilities, and I use them to their full potential.

You aren't being delusional or ignoring reality when you replace your negative thoughts with healthier, positive ones. You are simply choosing to see the other side of the coin. It has been there all along; you just haven't been looking at it. There is more than one way to think about every situation and event in your life. When you choose to see the positive, you are agreeing with God's perspective—you are agreeing with his view of you, your circumstances, and the people he has put around you. That alone will propel you toward a fuller, happier life. As Paul wrote:

> *God is in the process of transforming you, but he can't complete that work in you unless you let him, unless you cooperate with him by letting his thoughts become your thoughts*

Don't copy the behavior and customs of this world, but *let God transform you into a new person by changing the way you think.* Then you will learn to know God's will for you, which is good and pleasing and perfect. (Rom. 12:2, emphasis added)

There it is. God is in the process of transforming you, but he can't complete that work in you unless you let him, unless you cooperate with him by letting his thoughts become your thoughts.

185

Do your part to step out of your old ingrained thinking, the thinking that has left you feeling less than what you know you can be, and fill your mind instead with thoughts that can raise you to the best, truest version of yourself—the new you, ready to accept the abundant life God has in store for you (John 10:10).

Small Steps to the New You

1. Be intentional about listening to your internal monologue.

2. When you catch yourself having a negative or self-defeating thought, immediately replace it with a healthier thought.

3. Commit to memorizing one Scripture verse every week. Write it down and tape it to your bathroom mirror. Start with this one:

   Fix your thoughts on what is true, and honorable, and right, and pure, and lovely, and admirable. Think about things that are excellent and worthy of praise. (Phil. 4:8)

19

renewing your mind

The Powerful Effects of Prayer and How to Do It

A sound mind in a sound body, is a short, but full description of a happy state in this world: he that has these two, has little more to wish for; and he that wants either of them, will be little the better for anything else.

John Locke

Let God transform you into a new person by changing the way you think. Then you will learn to know God's will for you, which is good and pleasing and perfect.

Romans 12:2

Sometimes when my husband, Brian, and I (Jennifer) are talking with another person or another couple, I notice that he and I have a tendency to say the same thing, in the same way, at the same time. For example, if someone is telling a story, we often interject an "uh-huh" at the same time or react with the same phrase when the story is over. As scary as that may sound, it is completely natural. When you spend as much time with another person as we spend together, you begin to pick up their words, their phrasing, and even their tonality. Early on in a close relationship, you may find yourself using words you have never used before simply because the person you have been spending so much time with uses them. They get in your ear, and it doesn't take long to start adopting them as your own.

This reality goes a long way toward proving the old idiom: "You are the same today as you'll be in five years except for two things—the people you associate with and the books you read." What you allow into your mind is critical to your ongoing health and well-being. You become like the people you spend the most time with. The people you talk to the most influence what you say when you talk to yourself and to others. So you should be extremely choosy about the people your most frequent conversations are with. Those conversations—whether they are with a spouse, a close friend, or a coworker—will greatly influence the direction of your life over time.

Given the weight of this truth, here is an idea to consider: What if the person you talked to the most was God? What if, as you moved through your day, you were engaged in an ongoing dialogue with him? Not in a weird, kneel-down-in-the-lunch-line kind of way but rather in simple, quiet thoughts directed toward him and an intentional focus on hearing what he might want to say to you in return. Or to put it another way, what if you engaged in ongoing prayer? Those conversations with God would begin to shape the way you think, the way you speak to yourself, and the way you approach your life.

Prayer is key for your ongoing mental clarity and strength. It renews your mind and allows God to change the way you see the world. And the good news is that prayer isn't complicated. Prayer is simply talking with God, telling him what is going on with you and being quiet long enough to hear from him. When you make

spending time in communication with God
a habit, his truth will begin to saturate your
mind. Your thinking will shift so it is more in
line with his. The time you spend with him
will begin to have an effect on you, just as any

*Prayer is key for your
ongoing mental
clarity and strength.*

ongoing influence does. And what better influence to be affected
by? Prayer really works; it not only changes circumstances but also
changes you—physically, spiritually, emotionally, and mentally.

A well-renowned cardiologist at Duke University Medical Center once became intrigued by the notion of prayer's ability to alter
outcomes and decided to do an experiment on his heart patients.
He set out, asking the question, *Is there a measurable, incremental
benefit to prayer?* After the experiment ended, the doctor provided
his conclusion on an interview with the Discovery Channel:

> We saw impressive reductions in all of the negative outcomes of
> heart patients. . . . What we look for routinely in cardiology trials are outcomes such as death, heart attack, or lungs filling with
> water—what we call congestive heart failure. . . . In the group randomly assigned prayer therapy, there was 50 percent reduction in all
> complications and a 100 percent reduction in major complications.[1]

In an unrelated study, a physician at the Pacific College of Medicine in San Francisco set out to test the effect of prayer on advanced
AIDS patients. Her findings were similar. She discovered that the
patients who received prayer had six times fewer hospitalizations
than the people who received no prayer, and those hospitalizations were significantly shorter. She said in an interview, "I was
shocked. In a way, it was like witnessing a miracle. There is no
way to understand this from my experience, from my basic understanding of science."[2]

When asked to comment on this and other similar medical
studies, the late Chuck Colson, a prominent Christian observer
of culture, said, "Such studies have plenty of critics, but the new

research has left many scratching their heads. Is prayer something that can be put under a microscope and examined? Probably not. But one thing is for sure, prayer works and prayer is real."[3]

Though science will likely never be able to define exactly what happens in our conversations with God, one thing is for sure: they have significant effects on our health and well-being.

Communicating with God

Stop and think about the incredible privilege of prayer for a minute. You have the ability to communicate with God—the author of the world, your Creator—whenever and wherever you want. You don't have to know a secret code, use any particular phrasing, or go through a priest. You can talk with God anytime. He is ready and willing to engage in conversation with you. In fact, he wants you to make talking to him a regular part of your day. As Paul wrote, "Devote yourselves to prayer with an alert mind and a thankful heart" (Col. 4:2).

When you immerse yourself in conversation with God, you do three things that act as catalysts for aligning your mind with his. When you talk to God, you

- acknowledge his existence;
- connect with him on a deeper level; and
- demonstrate your dependence on him.

Acknowledge His Existence

When you pray, you demonstrate your belief in God's existence. Ninety percent of Americans say they believe God is real. Out of the 90 percent, over 50 percent pray on a regular basis.[4] That 50 percent is proving what they say they believe. To them, God isn't just a concept or a question mark. He is an actual being they can engage with. Their actions give credence to their belief and acknowledge the tangible existence of God himself.

Interestingly, the 10 percent who say they don't believe in God help to prove his existence just as powerfully as those who engage in regular prayer. While they may spend decades in debates trying to disprove the existence of a higher power (atheists) or contending that there is no way to know if there is a God (agnostics), self-proclaimed nonbelievers are quick to pray to the one they disavow when tragedy strikes. As the old saying goes, "There are no atheists in foxholes." When the temporal is in turmoil, something inside every human being cries out for the eternal. We are wired for a connection with our Creator. It is crucial to our well-being.

Connect with Him on a Deeper Level

Your relationship with God, if you are a Christian, is a bit like your relationship with your spouse, if you are married. On your wedding day, you stood in front of your family and friends and made a lifelong commitment to the person you love. You and your husband or wife to be recited vows, pledging to honor and cherish each other, had some cake, and then set out on your new life together. But then what? Did you stop talking to each other after the wedding was over? Of course not. If you had, your marriage would have crumbled more quickly than that cake. Instead, you started engaging in an ongoing conversation that creates a healthy married life.

So it is with God. An initial connection with God happens when you submit your life to him, when you allow him to move into the core of your being and take control. But that connection is just the beginning. God wants to continually deepen the relationship as you choose to engage him in conversation through daily prayer. Your prayers have the ability to move you into his presence and to put you in a position to hear what he wants to say to you.

191

Demonstrate Your Dependence on Him

I (Nelson) have an engineer friend who, as part of his job, regularly oversees the development of large residential buildings in different parts of the country. Every time he starts a new project, he spends an incredible amount of time with the architect who designed the building. They go over plans and blueprints together ad nauseam. There is no way my friend would begin a new building project without being crystal clear on what the designer had in mind. That would be crazy. If he failed to follow the blueprints of the person with the complete vision for the job, disaster would be right around the corner.

Even so, that is how millions of people go about building their lives. They forge ahead with what they think is in their best interest, neglecting to consult the One who has the blueprint. But there is no reason to barrel ahead blindly. By choosing to communicate with God every day, you place yourself in a position where he can show you the best possible plan for your life and give you what you need to live it out.

Let me be clear, though. Prayer is not ultimately about God being available to you. It is about you being available to God. It is about letting him know that you are ready and willing for him to shape your life. As you admit your dependence on him and acknowledge that his plan is bigger and better than your own, you open the door for him to work in your life. Some of the most powerful, most life-transforming words you can ever speak are, "God, I need you. Please show me the path you want me to walk." God won't force himself on you, but if you will engage in the conversation, he will be sure to carry his end of it.

Something to Talk About

Don't you hate it when you are trying to talk to someone but you don't really have anything to say? Or when you stumble into one of those awkward lulls in the conversation so big it could swallow a house? Some people never have that problem, but those of you who are a little more introverted can probably relate.

Many people admit that this is their hang-up with talking to God—they just don't know where to begin. A loss for words with God stems from an incorrect view of who he is and what he expects from us. We become stagnated when we feel as if we need to impress him or feel that we can't be ourselves—but neither of those things should apply to our conversations with the One who created us. He already knows everything about us, so there is no reason to approach him with anything other than complete transparency.

> *A loss for words with God stems from an incorrect view of who he is and what he expects from us.*

While teaching a group of disciples how to pray, Jesus emphasized that we don't have to approach God with anything other than who we are. God doesn't want us to go to him putting on airs, using high, theological language and trying to talk about things we aren't really interested in. He is simply looking for an earnest conversation. Matthew 6:5–6 says:

> When you pray, don't be like the hypocrites who love to pray publicly on street corners and in the synagogues where everyone can see them. I tell you the truth, that is all the reward they will ever get. But when you pray, go away by yourself, shut the door behind you, and pray to your Father in private.

God wants you to approach him simply. Once you realize that, you can get down to the business of being yourself and having open, honest conversations with him about the things that are bothering you, the things you need help with, the things you need to hand over to him, and the list goes on. The more you talk to God and place your dependence on him, the healthier your mind will become.

Praying for Yourself

See if you can relate to this scenario. It is five minutes before a big presentation, an important conversation, or a major event, and you find yourself praying, "Oh, God, please be with me here. This is such a big deal, and it really needs to go well. If you could just supernaturally intervene right now, I would be grateful." Then as an afterthought, you say, "Oh, and help those who need you around the world, and be with my brother while he travels. Amen." Does that kind of prayer resonate?

If you tend to pray selfish prayers, you are not alone. We all like to talk about ourselves to God—what we want, what we need, what we think he can do to help us. And here is the good news: God is okay with those kinds of prayers. David wrote, "In the day when I cried out, You answered me, and made me bold with strength in my soul" (Ps. 138:3 NKJV).

God wants you to go to him with every need, no matter how large or small. He will answer you. He will calm your mind. He will give you comfort and peace. Now, if every one of your prayers sounded like the one above, that wouldn't be good, but there is nothing wrong with praying for yourself. As you do, make sure you pray confidently, boldly, humbly, and faithfully.

Pray Confidently

God is for you. He loves you and wants to give you good things. He wants your life to have maximum impact and fulfillment. When you pray, pray with the confidence that comes along with that reality. Don't expect anything less than God's best. Know that your prayers will be heard and answered because you are his child. Look at what Jesus said:

> You parents—if your children ask for a loaf of bread, do you give them a stone instead? Or if they ask for a fish, do you give them a snake? Of course not! So if you sinful people know how to give

194

good gifts to your children, how much more will your heavenly Father give good gifts to those who ask him. (Matt. 7:9–11)

Good parents build their children up and encourage them. They focus on their children's strengths rather than their faults and do their best to provide them with everything they need.

In the same way, when God looks at you, he is not fixated on your flaws or focused on your deficiencies. Rather, he is proud of you, fiercely protective of you, and focused on helping you live the abundant life he has in store. Why? Simply because he is your heavenly Father and you are his child. When you are walking in that truth, you can approach God with renewed confidence, knowing that he is for you and working everything together for your good.

Pray Boldly

Too many of us are inclined to pray meek, tentative prayers. We figure that what we have to say probably isn't important enough to bother God with; we assume he has more pressing issues at hand. But the Bible tells us over and over again that if we are followers of Jesus, we should pray boldly, expecting God to answer us. Jesus said it this way: "You can ask for anything in my name, and I will do it" (John 14:13).

Have you ever wondered why you have to ask God for the things you need? After all, if he knows everything about you, he already knows what you need. Why does he make you go through the process of asking? Just think about it: If God gave you everything you wanted or needed before you even asked, how would you know that the good things in your life were coming from him?

Often, when people stop talking with God regularly, they begin to see the circumstances in their lives that are actually blessings from God as random chance or luck. Sometimes they begin to take credit for the good they are experiencing; they miss the evidence of

God's hand because they weren't talking to him about their needs and wants on the front end. But when you ask God for something specific and then that specific thing comes to pass, you know beyond the shadow of a doubt where it came from. God will get the glory, praise, and credit he deserves.

Praying boldly is simply praying with the aforementioned confidence that God hears your prayers and wants to bless you. Bold prayers garner big responses. As Jesus said, "I tell you the truth, if you have faith and don't doubt, you can do things like this and much more. You can even say to this mountain, 'May you be lifted up and thrown into the sea,' and it will happen. You can pray for anything, and if you have faith, you will receive it" (Matt. 21:21–22). Faith and doubt cannot coexist. So pray boldly for the job you are applying for. Pray boldly for the child you want to come into your marriage. Pray boldly for healing in the health situation you are dealing with. Pray boldly that God will bless you in the areas where you need blessing. No matter the situation or what you are praying for, use bold words. God will hear them and answer you accordingly.

Pray Humbly

At first glance, you may consider it contradictory to approach God with confident boldness and with humility at the same time, but there is no contradiction at all. Being humble before God simply means acknowledging that God is God and you are not. When you talk to him, use bold and confident words, but do so from a place of humility that shows you submit to his ultimate will.

When a child comes to a parent and asks for something that isn't in their best interest, a loving parent says no, even if the child asks with confidence and boldness. The same is true with God. If you are praying for something that is outside his will for your life, he won't answer in the way you expect. With humility, trust that he knows more than you do; he sees farther than you can see.

Bold, confident prayers don't force God to do anything. They usher in his blessing when they are in line with his will for your life, but they don't manipulate him into giving you something that is out of alignment with his ultimate goals for you. The greater purpose of talking with God through prayer is to line up your wants and needs with his will and desires—to have your thoughts renewed by aligning them with his.

Pray Faithfully

You cannot approach God with the confidence, boldness, and humility he desires if your conversations with him aren't rooted in a foundation of faith. He has promised to hear and answer the prayers of those who have placed their trust in him, but he has not promised the same to those yet to profess their belief. Sometimes he will answer the prayer of an unbeliever for one of two reasons: (1) to bring glory to himself or (2) to help move that person toward a relationship with him—but he makes no promises to answer. There is one prayer, however, that God will always answer. That is the earnest prayer of someone choosing to put their faith in him for the first time. For more about stepping into a faith relationship with God, go to NewYouBook.com.

Praying for Others

While connecting with God about what is going on in our lives is crucial to our continued mental well-being, talking to him about others is also key. Since so many of our worries and frustrations involve other people, we can find relief by praying for and about our family members, friends, coworkers, and anyone else who may be weighing heavily on our minds. Here are a few reasons why praying for other people is important:

- *God says to pray for other people.* Part of loving others well is being willing to go to God on their behalf, which takes both time and intentionality. Richard Foster, a philosopher on prayer, writes, "If we truly love people we will desire for them far more than is within our power to give them and this will lead us to prayer."[5] Intercession gives you the ability to influence other people's lives in substantial ways.

- *Praying for other people grows your faith.* When you pray for someone and God answers that prayer, your faith increases. Praying for others is good for your own spiritual health.

- *Praying for others strengthens relationships.* Praying for someone draws you closer to that person. No matter where they are in the world—whether right next door to you or several continents away—you will feel more connected in the relationship because of your prayers. And you know how important strong relationships are to your overall health.

- *Praying for others impacts the world.* When you pray for another person, you are cooperating with God in helping that person become all they are meant to be. You are playing an important part in raising that person up to their full potential in Christ.

But what, specifically, should you pray for when you pray for other people? There are two types of prayers for others that should be on your lips often—one comes very naturally, while the other takes more perspective and intentionality. When you pray for the people in your life, focus on praying for safety and significance.

Praying for Others' Safety

Concern over the day-to-day safety and well-being of family and friends is natural for most of us. Still, when it comes to praying that your mother has a safe flight or that your friend's doctor's appointment goes well, you may be likely to think that God is too busy to be concerned, which can lead you to stop praying and simply hold your breath. Remember, God is never too busy to hear your cries to him, no matter how big or small they may seem. He is concerned with what concerns you, which means he is more than willing to hear and answer prayers about the safety of those you love. Handing those concerns over to him and trusting him for your loved ones' safety will allow you to let go of worry.

What does praying for safety look like, practically speaking? First of all, you should pray for overall protection for your loved ones. Then you can pray specifically for what is going on with each one. When you pray specific prayers, you will be able to see God answer those prayers and can celebrate accordingly. Maybe you pray for safe travels for a friend taking a long trip; maybe you pray protection over a family member who is dealing with a chronic health issue; perhaps your prayer is for a smooth recovery for someone you care about who has been sick or for

> *God is never too busy to hear your cries to him, no matter how big or small they may seem.*

your child's safety as they play competitive sports. Whatever safety issues you are concerned about, take them to God—and then leave them with him

Praying for Others' Significance

Moving things up a notch, you should also pray for significance for the people you love. That is, you should pray that their lives will be filled with substance and meaning, that they will make a difference in the world, that God's purposes will be done through them.

If you study prayer in Scripture, you will see that most prayers are more along these lines than they are focused on immediate concerns. In fact, Paul prayed some of the most powerful prayers of significance for others ever recorded. Take a look at this prayer for the believers in a town called Ephesus:

> I pray for you constantly, asking God, the glorious Father of our Lord Jesus Christ, to give you spiritual wisdom and insight so that you might grow in your knowledge of God. I pray that your hearts will be flooded with light so that you can understand the confident hope he has given to those he called—his holy people who are his rich and glorious inheritance. I also pray that you will understand the incredible greatness of God's power for us who believe him. This is the same mighty power that raised Christ from the dead and seated him in the place of honor at God's right hand in the heavenly realms. (Eph. 1:16–20)

What a prayer! Can you imagine what would happen in the lives of those around you if you were praying that kind of prayer over them every day? What would happen in your life if people were praying such a prayer over you? The details of everyday life often keep us so caught up in the mundane that we forget that we have access to the incredible resurrection power of Jesus within us.

Even as we pray for safe road trips and effective medical treatments, let's not neglect to pray for "spiritual wisdom and insight" and that the hearts of those we love will be "flooded with light so that they can understand the confident hope God has given them." Pray for your loved ones to be renewed by God, to be used by God, and to do God's will.

If you get into the practice of praying for safety and significance for the people you love, not only will you be making a tangible difference in their lives, but you will also begin seeing subtle shifts in how you interact with them. When you let your interactions with others grow out of your heartfelt conversations with God about them, your relationships will be strengthened and your family and friends will be influenced in ways you can only imagine.

Be Still

As you enter conversations with God, take time to be still and listen to what he has to say. Resist the urge to do all the talking. Just as in any conversation, there has to be give-and-take. Overtalking is one of the most common ways we block our ability to hear from God. Too often, our prayers go something like this, "God, if you will just show me the path I should take, I will take it. You are so good, God. You have been good to me in the past. I want to honor you. Let me know what I should do next. I am ready to hear from you. Amen." Then we get up, walk away, and question why God didn't speak to us during our prayer time. You have to wonder if God is in heaven thinking, *I would love to tell you my will for your life, but I can't get a word in edgewise!*

If only we could learn to listen better, we would have deeper conversations with God. As David wrote in Psalm 46, God wants us to "be still, and know that I am God!" (v. 10).

Being still in your conversations with God will allow you to get to know him more intimately, which has some practical benefits. Knowing God better will draw you deeper into the richness of life Jesus has promised—a life with more well-being, better health in every area, clearer purpose, and greater impact.

Small Steps to the New You

1. Set aside fifteen minutes to have a conversation with God.

2. Practice talking with God the way you would talk to a good friend. Don't feel as if you need to say anything specific. Just thank him for the good things in your life and tell him what you are worried about.

3. Be quick to turn your mind back toward God at various points throughout your day as things pop up that concern you or that you feel thankful for.

4. Visit NewYouBook.com to download some free resources on prayer.

conclusion

The glory of God is man fully alive.

St. Irenaeus

This means that anyone who belongs to Christ has become a new person. The old life is gone; a new life has begun!

2 Corinthians 5:17

The Chinese bamboo tree is an interesting, gorgeous tree that grows in the Far East. When farmers plant the seed for a Chinese bamboo tree, they know they are taking on a task that will require incredible patience. Every day for four years, they will water and fertilize the seed. During that time, there will be absolutely no visible growth. The seed will stay locked away underground, and it will look as though nothing is happening. Then in the fifth year, the consistent, small steps to ensure the tree's health will pay off. The tree will break through the soil and begin growing at an unbelievable rate. In just five weeks or so, it will grow to be ninety feet tall.

To gear up and get started, those tree farmers had to have a great deal of faith in the small steps of watering and fertilizing. They had to have a crystal clear understanding of the truth that you reap what you sow. And they had to have incredible patience, knowing that if they kept at it, their effort would pay off in a breathtaking, God-glorifying way.

The same is true for your health and wellness. But thankfully, you won't have to wait five years to see results. Many of the small steps we have outlined in these pages will lead to fast results, while some will require longer periods of consistent nurturing before they show themselves. But all the "Small Steps to the New You," when taken consistently over a period of time, will eventually lead to the growth of a life that will exceed your wildest dreams.

Fully Alive

When you enter a personal relationship with Jesus, as we have discussed in these pages, you are not just refreshed, reformed, or rehabilitated. You are not turning over a new leaf. You are not embarking on a self-help journey. Rather, you are transformed from the inside out—and not as a result of anything you have done or can do but because of what Jesus has done. Take another look at Paul's words, in a little more context:

> How differently we know him now! This means that anyone who belongs to Christ has become a new person. The old life is gone; a new life has begun! And all of this is a gift from God, who brought us back to himself through Christ. (2 Cor. 5:16–18)

Again, walking in the reality of your new life in Christ doesn't hinge on trying harder or doing better. It is about surrendering to the fullness of your new identity in him and doing your part to live out that fullness in every aspect of your daily life.

Choose to walk in the truth of who you are in Jesus every single day. Choose to take responsibility for your health and well-being in every area so that you can be an example of his goodness to an

onlooking world. Choose to be a good steward of the opportunities God has given you to love others completely and fulfill his
purposes. In other words, choose to water the seeds within you.
Then when you least expect it, you will realize that your outer life
has become an astounding reflection of the new creation you are
on the inside. You will be living in the reality of the new you. Here
are some final steps to help you get started.

Stop Procrastinating

Procrastination derails more good intentions than just about
anything else. We always think we can eat whatever we want to
today because we are going to start losing weight tomorrow. We
justify staying up late tonight because we can rest when there is
less going on. We put off having the hard conversation that could
heal a relationship because there is no point in starting an argument right now. Who's guilty?

The problem is that tomorrow always becomes today, and when
it does, something else inevitably gives us an excuse to wait until
the next tomorrow to get started. But the book of Proverbs warns,
"Don't brag about tomorrow, since you don't know what the day
will bring" (27:1). Tomorrow may bring circumstances that will
make doing what needs to be done even harder, or tomorrow may
actually be too late. Heart attacks happen in the blink of an eye.
Diagnoses come out of left field. There may be seedlings of diseases lurking inside you right now that have the potential to come
to fruition and overtake you if you continue to put off doing the
things that create health. You don't know when it is going to be
too late to turn back; you can't afford to keep procrastinating.

Invest in Yourself

You are committed to investing in others. You pour into your
family, your friends, your coworkers, and so many other people.

But how committed are you to investing in yourself? If you don't take the time to care for your own health and well-being, you will eventually lose your ability to be there for anyone else.

Don't fall into the trap of thinking that self-sacrifice to the point of physical, mental, and emotional exhaustion is a badge of honor. Yes, you have responsibilities to the people in your life. Yes, you are supposed to count others' interests ahead of your own. But you are also called to take care of yourself in a way that will allow you to continue doing those things effectively. Take a look at what Jesus had to say to his apostles when they were in a particularly busy season:

> The apostles returned to Jesus from their ministry tour and told him all they had done and taught. Then Jesus said, "Let's go off by ourselves to a quiet place and rest awhile." He said this because there were so many people coming and going that Jesus and his apostles didn't even have time to eat. (Mark 6:30–31)

If you don't take the time to take care of yourself—to "come apart," as some other biblical translations put it—you will soon come apart at the seams. Or as we like to say, if you don't come apart, you will come apart. Neglecting to invest in yourself by eating properly, moving your body, resting well, reducing stress, nurturing healthy relationships, and doing the other things required for health will destroy you and your ability to do all that God has given you to do.

I (Nelson) recently heard a story about a woman who called her church's office and asked to speak to the pastor. The secretary said, "I'm sorry, the pastor is not available. Today is his Sabbath. He'll be in tomorrow."

The following Sunday that woman marched up to the pastor, got right in his face, and said, "I really needed to talk to you last week, and your secretary said you were taking the day off! Satan doesn't take a day off!"

The pastor responded, "You are exactly right. He doesn't. And if I don't take a day off, I'm going to end up just like Satan." The same holds true for you. You have to care for yourself to be able to keep living and loving well.

Commit to a Healthy Lifestyle in All Four Areas

To choose new life, you must adopt a lifestyle that promotes and sustains life. As we have discussed at length, getting healthy physically, spiritually, emotionally, and mentally takes long-term thinking. Instead of giving in to the temptation to make a quick fix in any area, you must commit to an ongoing healthy lifestyle. The best way to determine whether the changes you are making can be part of such a lifestyle is to ask yourself, "Is this something I could continue doing for the rest of my life?" If the answer is no, you aren't developing a lifestyle; you are simply on a crash course. Reevaluate your approach.

> *You have to care for yourself to be able to keep living and loving well.*

Your healthy lifestyle won't look exactly like ours or anyone else's. Yes, there are universal rules about health that we all need to work within (as we have discussed), but the day-to-day specifics of what you eat, how you exercise, when you have your quiet time with God, how you make time to rest, and the like will be unique to you. Keep those specifics conducive to your long-range goals. Focus on small steps every day and watch your life transform.

Decide to Maximize Your Impact

God gave you life so that you can make a difference. Still, as believers, we don't always feel at home in this world. We long for the sweetness of heaven. As Paul wrote:

> I'm torn between two desires: I long to go and be with Christ, which would be far better for me. But for your sakes, it is better that I

continue to live. Knowing this, I am convinced that I will remain alive so I can continue to help all of you grow and experience the joy of your faith. (Phil. 1:23–25)

In this passage, Paul is essentially saying that he is choosing life, not just for his own benefit but so that he can positively influence those coming behind him.

In the same way, choose life so that you can impact those who have been placed in your path. People who choose to neglect their health, ending up sick and struggling to get through each day, rarely have much impact on the world. And dead people have even less. By deciding to get healthy, you are taking a major step toward maximizing the difference your life can make now and in generations to come.

Consider this passage: "Only take heed to yourself, and diligently keep yourself, lest you forget the things your eyes have seen, and lest they depart from your heart all the days of your life. And teach them to your children and your grandchildren" (Deut. 4:9 NKJV). Do you have children? Do you have grandchildren? Even if you don't right now, one day God may bless you with both. If that day comes, you owe it to them to be healthy and vibrant, ready and able to engage with them well. You owe it to yourself to be able to participate in their lives at full capacity for as long as possible. Being able to be with your loved ones for the long haul is much more significant than the few minutes of enjoyment you get out of that greasy hamburger, the sweat you avoid by not exercising, or the little bit more work you get done by refusing to rest.

Short-term pleasures and easier paths aren't worth missing out on lasting memories with your family.

The things that rob you of your health are so often the same things that rob you of your potential to live and love well—and they are just not worth it. They never will be. Short-term pleasures and easier paths aren't worth missing out on lasting memories with

207

your family. And they aren't worth missing out on the plans God has for your one, wonderful life.

Living for Today, Tomorrow, and Eternity

One day—on the day you leave this world for your home in heaven—you will receive a glorified body. As Scripture teaches, there will be no more pain and no more suffering (Rev. 21:4). You will be whole and eternally healthy. What a glorious day that will be, as the old hymn says. But until that day comes, you have a responsibility to take care of the earthly vessel God has given you in a way that reveals his excellence, to make it an example of honor and strength, capable of accomplishing the purposes he has for you.

Our prayer is that, with God's help, you will make daily choices that will allow this to happen. Choose to live in a way that will allow you to experience the abundance God offers today, to impact the people around you for a better tomorrow, and to alter eternity in a positive way forevermore.

Friend, it is time to take responsibility for your health. It is time to take responsibility for your life. Are you ready? Don't settle for being tired, stressed, foggy, sick, and overweight. Don't let anyone or anything convince you that you are capable of only second best in the areas that matter most.

God has given you strength; nurture it. He has given you vitality; protect it. He has given you opportunity; stay well so you can fulfill it. Choose to step away from the masses and live a better life. Choose to walk fully in the new life that God gave you when you gave yourself to him. As you do, he will be able to do more in you and through you than you have ever imagined.

> Now all glory to God, who is able, through his mighty power at work within us, to accomplish infinitely more than we might ask or think. Glory to him in the church and in Christ Jesus through all generations forever and ever! Amen. (Eph. 3:20–21)

Small Steps to the New You

1. Decide to stop procrastinating. Make a point to eat something healthy and do some type of exercise today. Get to bed earlier tonight. Offer someone forgiveness.

2. Look back through the "Small Steps to the New You" at the end of each chapter. Write down the ones you want to begin implementing right away.

3. Think about the person or people who motivate you to live a healthier, more complete life. Is it your spouse? Your children? Your grandchildren? Put a picture of that person or those people in a place where you will see it often. Focus on getting and staying healthy in every way so you can be fully present in your relationship with them for as long as possible.

4. Spend some time reflecting on all you have learned in these pages. Ask God to direct you and show you his grace as you begin living fully in the reality of the new you.

We hope this book will be the beginning of an ongoing conversation. Please visit NewYouBook.com to connect with us, access many free resources, and share your story.

the small steps challenge

This four-month plan will help you incorporate the "Small Steps to the New You" into your life in a strategic way. Start by reading the introduction through chapter 3. Then make the following three commitments before you dive into the four-month challenge. These three commitments form the foundation for your journey to complete health in Christ.

Surrender your health to God.
Begin by praying a prayer like this one:

> Dear God, I know that you made me. You created my body, my soul, and my spirit. You created me for your glory. I am sorry for the ways I have mistreated myself in the past. I am sorry for the excuses I have made for poor health choices and poor habits. I give this path to health and wholeness over to you. Please walk it with me. Please keep me focused on your truth, and help me to choose excellence every day. Thank you for creating me to live an abundant life, to do good work, and to love others well all my days. I surrender every aspect of my health to you now. Thank you for all you are going to do in and through me. Amen.

Stop making excuses.
What is the biggest excuse you make for why you are not where you want to be? Be honest with yourself. Don't be afraid to look

that excuse in the face. When you know what it is, refuse to make that excuse anymore. If you find it creeping into your mind, stop the thought and replace it with the following: God is able to do a great work in me.

Start taking small steps toward change.
Just picking up this book is a great step in the right direction. Tell someone you trust that you are reading it. Ask that person to hold you accountable to making healthy changes in your life.

Once you have made these three commitments, you are ready to start your journey to the new you. Over the next four months, you will begin making small changes in the four primary areas of health—physical health, spiritual health, emotional health, and mental health—one area and one month at a time.

Month 1: Small Steps to Better Physical Health
Month 2: Small Steps to Better Spiritual Health
Month 3: Small Steps to Better Emotional Health
Month 4: Small Steps to Better Mental Health

Each month work to incorporate as many small steps into your life as you can. Go at your own pace. Some of these steps will be quick and easy, and some will take more work. By the end of each month, you should be taking as many of that month's small steps as possible, as consistently as possible.

Month 1: Small Steps to Better Physical Health

- Take a hard look at the gluttonous habits you may have in your life. Decide to stop justifying them.

- Acknowledge that God's understanding of your physical health needs surpasses your own.
- Go to NewYouBook.com and listen to a message about breaking free from gluttony.
- Add more colorful fruits and vegetables into a few of your meals each week.
- Start reading nutrition labels on breads, pastas, and baked goods. Buy only products that are 100 percent whole grain.
- Trade white rice for brown rice.
- Try limiting your intake of meat to one meal a day.
- Acknowledge the reality of resistance in your life—and resist it!
- Take a ten-minute pause before snacking to make sure you are actually hungry.
- Claim a corner of the refrigerator for your healthy groceries.
- Choose restaurants that will have healthy options. You may even want to look at the menu online before you go so you know what your choices will be before you get there.
- Drink half your body weight in water every day. Divide your weight by two. That is how many ounces of water you should aim for on a daily basis. (For tips on how to drink more water throughout the day, see the "Small Steps to the New You" section in chapter 7.)
- Download a pedometer app or buy a pedometer to track the number of steps you are walking in a day. Try to hit ten thousand.
- Download a podcast or the audio version of a book you have been meaning to read and listen while you walk or work out.
- Put your workout clothes and sneakers by the bed the night before and take a morning walk as soon as you wake up.
- Need to call your mom? Plug some earbuds into your phone and take a walk around the neighborhood while you talk.

Month 2: Small Steps to Better Spiritual Health

- Take the quiz in chapter 9. Evaluate your answers. Jot down some ideas for how you could improve on each point.
- Think about this question: Who is Jesus? If you don't know the answer, decide to find out. Don't rely on your past experiences or what people tell you. Do your own intellectually honest research about his life and ministry.
- Seek out a healthy, Bible-based church in your area.
- Commit to being in church every weekend, as much as possible.
- Take one step toward deeper engagement with your church.
- Make a list of the supportive friends in your life. How many do you have? How authentic are these relationships?
- Seek out information about small groups at your church.
- Sign up for a small group and go!
- Choose to be aware of the needs around you.
- Act on small opportunities that present themselves daily.
- Pay attention to your passions and gifting and use them to serve others.

Month 3: Small Steps to Better Emotional Health

- Do the What-Went-Well exercise (chapter 13) before you go to bed each night, all month long.
- When you feel tempted to complain, find something positive to say instead.
- Have lunch or dinner with a friend from your small group and ask them about the good things going on in their life.
- Find a Christian counselor in your area and establish a relationship.

- Look over yesterday's to-do list. Put a plus sign next to every activity that filled you with energy and a minus sign next to what drained you. Going forward, try to focus more of your attention on the things that are a plus.
- Take fifteen minutes to declutter and organize your desk or one room in your home. If you think you can't finish in fifteen minutes, start anyway—and then do fifteen more minutes tomorrow.
- Put on some praise music and sing along while you make breakfast or run errands.
- Ask God to help you identify specific areas of bitterness in your heart.
- Make a list of the people you need to forgive and pray for the strength to do so.
- Forgive one person who hurt you using the process for biblical forgiveness (chapter 15). Then another person. Then another.
- Get out in the yard and do some weeding (if the season permits). It will solidify the image of uprooting bitterness—and give you some exercise to boot!
- Go to bed fifteen minutes earlier every night this month.
- Invest in a better mattress or begin saving up to buy one in the future.
- Try sleeping with a pillow between your knees to alleviate back pain.

Month 4: Small Steps to Better Mental Health

- Remind yourself as often as necessary that stress is a natural, unavoidable part of life.
- Make your to-do list either before you go to sleep at night or first thing in the morning.

- Practice eating frogs and living off peak. (See chapter 17.)
- When you are in a season that feels particularly stressful, set a timer every hour to remind you to think about the good in your life and to praise God for his faithfulness.
- Be intentional about listening to your internal monologue.
- When you catch yourself having a negative or self-defeating thought, immediately replace it with a healthier thought.
- Commit to memorizing one Scripture verse every week. Write it down and tape it to your bathroom mirror. Start with this one: "Fix your thoughts on what is true, and honorable, and right, and pure, and lovely, and admirable. Think about things that are excellent and worthy of praise" (Phil. 4:8).
- Set aside fifteen minutes to have a conversation with God each day this month.
- Practice talking with God the way you would talk to a good friend. Don't feel as if you need to say anything specific. Just thank him for the good things in your life and tell him what you are worried about.
- Be quick to turn your mind back toward God at various points throughout your day as things pop up that concern you or that you feel thankful for.
- Visit NewYouBook.com to download some free resources on prayer.
- Think about the person or people who motivate you to live a healthier, more complete life. Is it your spouse? Your children? Your grandchildren? Put a picture of that person or those people in a place where you will see it often. Focus on getting and staying healthy in every way so you can be fully present in your relationship with them for as long as possible.
- Spend some time reflecting on all you have learned over the last four months. Ask God to direct you and show you his grace as you begin living fully in the reality of the new you.

notes

Chapter 1 Whose You Are

1. Zig Ziglar, *Over the Top: Moving from Survival to Stability to Success, from Success to Significance* (Nashville: Thomas Nelson, 1997) loc. 3673, Kindle.

2. Rick Warren, Daniel Amen, and Mark Hyman, *The Daniel Plan: 40 Days to a Healthier Life* (Grand Rapids: Zondervan, 2013), 20.

Chapter 4 Your Secret Sin

1. Laurette Dube, *Obesity Prevention: The Role of Brain and Society on Individual Behavior* (Cambridge, MA: Academic Press, 2010), 654.

2. Rex Russell, *What the Bible Says about Healthy Living*, 2nd ed. (Ventura, CA: Regal, 2006), 37.

Chapter 5 Eating for Life

1. Jordan Rubin, *The Maker's Diet* (New York: Penguin, 2004), 31.

2. Joel Fuhrman, *Eat to Live: The Amazing Nutrient-Rich Program for Fast and Sustained Weight Loss*, rev. ed. (New York: Little, Brown, 2011), 82.

3. Fuhrman, *Eat to Live*, 88.

4. J. Salmeron et al., "Dietary Fiber, Glycemic Load, and Risk of NIDDM in Men," *US National Library of Medicine* 1 (April 1997), https://www.ncbi.nlm.nih.gov/pubmed/9096978.

5. "National Diabetes Statistics Report, 2014," Centers for Disease Control and Prevention, October 24, 2014, www.cdc.gov/diabetes/pdfs/data/2014-report-estimates-of-diabetes-and-its-burden-in-the-united-states.pdf.

6. Fuhrman, *Eat to Live*, 50.

7. Fuhrman, *Eat to Live*, 114.

8. Fuhrman, *Eat to Live*, 115.

Chapter 6 Avoiding Common Obstacles

1. Steven Pressfield, *Do the Work! Overcome Resistance and Get Out of Your Own Way* (Hastings, NY: Do You Zoom, 2011), 6, 8–9.

Chapter 7 Drink Up

1. "Health Challenge Week 3: Why Drinking Water Is Important for Weight Loss," *Central Wellness* (blog), May 3, 2018, https://centralwellness.com/health-challenge/drinking-water-is-important-for-weight-loss/.
2. Don Colbert, *The Seven Pillars of Health: The Natural Way to Better Health for Life* (Lake Mary, FL: Charisma Media, 2007), 31.

Chapter 8 Made to Move

1. Chris Kresser, "How Sitting Too Much Is Making Us Sick and Fat—and What to Do about It," *Huffington Post*, April 8, 2013, https://chriskresser.com/how-sitting-too-much-is-making-us-sick-and-fat-and-what-to-do-about-it/.
2. James H. Rimmer, PhD, "Sedentary Lifestyle Is Dangerous to Your Health," NCHPAD, accessed February 25, 2018, https://www.nchpad.org/403/2216/Sedentary~Lifestyle~is~Dangerous~to~Your~Health.
3. Steve Reynolds, personal communication, September 2014.
4. Jordan Rubin, *The Maker's Diet* (New York: Penguin, 2004), 174.
5. "Sitting Disease Is Taking a Toll on Your Body," Lifespan, April 4, 2013, https://www.lifespanfitness.com/workplace/resources/articles/sitting-all-day-is-taking-a-toll-on-your-body.

Chapter 9 Living the Fully Engaged Life

1. Albert L. Winseman, "How to Measure Spiritual Commitment," Gallup, April 30, 2012, https://news.gallup.com/poll/5914/how-measure-spiritual-commitment.aspx.

Chapter 10 Getting Connected

1. T. M. Luhrmann, "The Benefits of Church," *New York Times*, April 10, 2013, www.nytimes.com/2013/04/21/opinion/sunday/luhrmann-why-going-to-church-is-good-for-you.html.

Chapter 11 Finding Good Friends

1. Jane E. Brody, "Shaking Off Loneliness," *New York Times*, May 13, 2013, https://well.blogs.nytimes.com/2013/05/13/shaking-off-loneliness/.
2. Mega Ray, "Loneliness Linked to Alzheimer's Disease," *The Sunrise Blog*, November 5, 2015, www.sunriseseniorliving.com/blog/november-2015/loneliness-linked-to-alzheimers-disease.aspx.
3. Jane E. Brody, "The Surprising Effects of Loneliness on Health," *New York Times*, December 11, 2017, www.nytimes.com/2017/12/11/well/mind/how-loneliness-affects-our-health.html.

4. Stephanie Pappas, "7 Ways Friendships Are Great for Your Health," Live Science, January 8, 2016, www.livescience.com/53315-how-friendships-are-good-for-your-health.html.

Chapter 12 The Power of Serving

1. Leslie Goldman, "4 Amazing Health Benefits of Helping Others," *Huffington Post*, December 6, 2017, www.huffingtonpost.com/2013/12/28/health-benefits-of-helping-others_n_4427697.html.

2. "Unchurched Report: Survey of 2,000 Unchurched Americans," LifeWay Research, accessed February 26, 2018, http://lifewayresearch.com/wp-content/uploads/2017/01/BGCE-Unchurched-Study-Final-Report-1_5_17.pdf.

3. Andy Stanley as quoted in "#OC16: Save a Life, Andy Stanley," Slingshot Group, April 28, 2016, http://slingshotgroup.org/oc16-save-life-andy-stanley/.

Chapter 13 Managing Your Emotions

1. Melinda Smith et al., "Building Better Mental Health," HelpGuide.org, last updated March 2018, https://www.helpguide.org/articles/mental-health/building-better-mental-health.htm.

2. "Mind/Body Connection: How Your Emotions Affect Your Health," Family Doctor.org, last updated June 7, 2017, https://familydoctor.org/mindbody-connection-how-your-emotions-affect-your-health/.

3. Martin Seligman, PhD, *Flourish: A Visionary New Understanding of Happiness and Well-being* (New York: Atria Paperback, 2011), 33.

4. Seligman, *Flourish*, 33–34.

Chapter 15 Defeating the Deadliest Emotion

1. Sylvain-Jacques Desjardins, "Can Blaming Others Make People Sick?," Concordia University, August 9, 2011, http://www.concordia.ca/cunews/main/releases/2011/08/09/can-blaming-others-make-people-sick.html.

Chapter 16 The Sleep Connection

1. Arianna Huffington, *The Sleep Revolution: Transforming Your Life One Night at a Time* (New York: Harmony Books, 2017), 11.

2. Maggie Jones, "How Little Sleep Can You Get Away With?," *New York Times*, April 15, 2011, https://www.nytimes.com/2011/04/17/magazine/mag-17-Sleep-t.html.

3. Jeffrey M. Jones, "In U.S., 40% Get Less Than Recommended Amount of Sleep," Gallup, December 19, 2013, http://news.gallup.com/poll/166553/less-recommended-amount-sleep.aspx.

4. Huffington, *The Sleep Revolution*, 27.

5. R. Morgan Griffin, "9 Surprising Reasons to Get More Sleep," WebMD, last updated December 27, 2011, https://www.webmd.com/sleep-disorders/features/9-reasons-to-sleep-more#1.

6. Huffington, *The Sleep Revolution*, 28.

7. Huffington, *The Sleep Revolution*, 8.

Chapter 17 Sidestepping Stress

1. "Stress Symptoms: Effects of Stress on the Body," WebMD, accessed March 28, 2018, https://www.webmd.com/balance/stress-management/stress-symptoms -effects_of-stress-on-the-body#1.

Chapter 18 The Voice in Your Head

1. James Allen, *As a Man Thinketh* (West Valley City, UT: Waking Lion, 2007), 10.
2. Shad Helmstetter, *What to Say When You Talk to Yourself* (New York: Pocket Books, 1987), 62–71.
3. Allen, *As a Man Thinketh*, 13.
4. Stephen R. Covey, *The 7 Habits of Highly Effective People* (Provo, UT: Franklin Covey, 1998), 99–103.
5. Covey, *The 7 Habits of Highly Effective People*, 100.
6. Norman Vincent Peale, *The Power of Positive Thinking* (New York: Prentice-Hall, 1952), 46.
7. Helmstetter, *What to Say When You Talk to Yourself*, 85–87.

Chapter 19 Renewing Your Mind

1. Nathan Bupp, "Follow-Up Study on Prayer Therapy May Help Refute False and Misleading Information about Earlier Clinical Trial," Skeptic, July 22, 2005, www.skeptic.com/eskeptic/05-09-02/.
2. Chuck Colson, "Can Prayer Heal?," BreakPoint, October 12, 2001, http://www.breakpoint.org/2001/10/can-prayer-heal/.
3. Colson, "Can Prayer Heal?"
4. Frank Newport, "Most Americans Still Believe in God," Gallup, June 29, 2016, https://news.gallup.com/poll/193271/americans-believe-god.aspx; Michael Lipka, "5 Facts about prayer," FactTank, Pew Research Center, May 4, 2016, http://www.pewresearch.org/fact-tank/2016/05/04/5-facts-about-prayer/.
5. Richard Foster, *Prayer: Finding the Heart's True Home—10th Anniversary Edition*, large print (New York: Harper Large Prints, 1992), 249.

Nelson Searcy is the founding and lead pastor of The Journey Church. He is the author of many bestselling books, including *The Generosity Ladder, Maximize, Connect, Ignite,* and *Launch.* He is the founder of ChurchLeaderInsights.com and the Renegade Pastors Network. Searcy lives with his wife and son in Boca Raton, Florida.

Jennifer Dykes Henson is a writer, wife, and mom to two young girls. She has coauthored several bestselling books, including *The Generosity Ladder* and *Tongue Pierced.* Previously, Jennifer worked with Dr. Charles Stanley as the marketing communications manager for In Touch Ministries. She lives with her family in Atlanta, Georgia.

Also Available

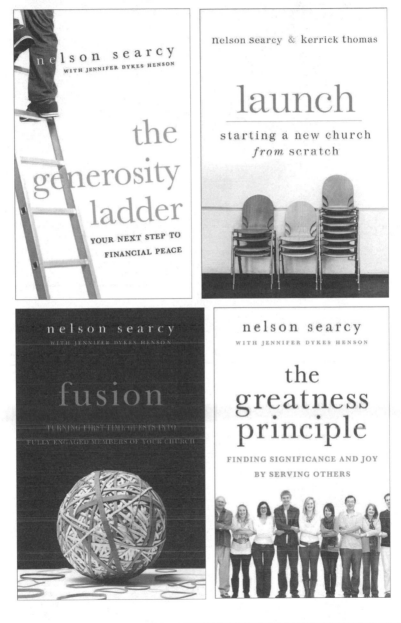

Connect with

DISCARDED BY
CAPITAL AREA DISTRICT LIBRARIES

Sign up for announcements about new and upcoming titles at

www.bakerbooks.com/signup

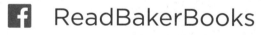 ReadBakerBooks

ReadBakerBooks